Resuscitation

Editor

JUSTIN DILIBERO

CRITICAL CARE NURSING CLINICS OF NORTH AMERICA

www.ccnursing.theclinics.com

Consulting Editor
CYNTHIA BAUTISTA

September 2021 • Volume 33 • Number 3

ELSEVIER

1600 John F. Kennedy Boulevard ● Suite 1800 ● Philadelphia, Pennsylvania, 19103-2899

http://www.theclinics.com

CRITICAL CARE NURSING CLINICS OF NORTH AMERICA Volume 33, Number 3
September 2021 ISSN 0899-5885, ISBN-13: 978-0-323-83602-9

Editor: Kerry Holland
Developmental Editor: Ann Gielou M. Posedio

Critical Care Nursing Clinics of North America (ISSN 0899-5885) is published quarterly by Elsevier Inc., 360 Park Avenue South, New York, NY 10010-1710. Months of issue are March, June, September, and December. Business and Editorial Offices: 1600 John F. Kennedy Blvd., Suite 1800, Philadelphia, PA 19103-2899. Periodicals postage paid at New York, NY and additional mailing offices. Subscription prices are $160.00 per year for US individuals, $576.00 per year for US institutions, $100.00 per year for US students and residents, $206.00 per year for Canadian individuals, $596.00 per year for Canadian institutions, $230.00 per year for international individuals, $596.00 per year for international institutions, $115.00 per year for international students/residents and $100.00 per year for Canadian students/residents. To receive student/resident rate, orders must be accompanied by name of affiliated institution, data of term, and the *signature* of program/residency coordinator on institution letterhead. Orders will be billed at individual rate until proof of status is received. Foreign air speed delivery is included in all *Clinics* subscription prices. All prices are subject to change without notice. **POSTMASTER:** Send address changes to *Critical Care Nursing Clinics of North America*, Elsevier Health Sciences Division, Subscription Customer Service, 3251 Riverport Lane, Maryland Heights, MO 63043. **Customer Service: 1-800-654-2452 (US and Canada); 314-447-8871 (outside US and Canada). Fax: 314-447-8029. E-mail:** JournalsCustomerService-usa@elsevier.com **(for print support) and** JournalsOnlineSupport-usa@elsevier.com **(for online support).**

Reprints. For copies of 100 or more of articles in this publication, please contact the Commercial Reprints Department, Elsevier Inc., 360 Park Avenue South, New York, New York, 10010-1710; Tel.: 212-633-3874, Fax: 212-633-3820, and E-mail: reprints@elsevier.com.

Critical Care Nursing Clinics of North America is covered in *MEDLINE/PubMed (Index Medicus), International Nursing Index, Nursing Citation Index, Cumulative Index to Nursing and Allied Health Literature, and RNdex Top 100.*

Contributors

CONSULTING EDITOR

CYNTHIA BAUTISTA, PhD, APRN, FNCS, FCNS
Associate Professor, Egan School of Nursing and Health Studies, Fairfield University, Fairfield, Connecticut

EDITOR

JUSTIN DILIBERO, DNP, APRN, CCRN-K, CCNS, ACCNS-AG, FCNS
Chair, Graduate Department, Director, Doctor of Nursing Practice Program, Assistant Professor, Rhode Island College School of Nursing, Rhode Island Nurse Education Center, Providence, Rhode Island

AUTHORS

AMANDA P. BETTENCOURT, PhD, APRN, CCRN-K, ACCNS-P
Research Fellow, Department of Systems, Populations, and Leadership, University of Michigan School of Nursing, Ann Arbor, Michigan

CAROLYN BRADLEY, MSN, RN, CCRN
Heart and Vascular Center Nursing Professional Development Specialist, Yale New Haven Hospital, New Haven, Connecticut

KRISTEN M. BURTON-WILLIAMS, MSN, APRN, ACCNS-AG, CCRN-K, TCRN, FCNS
Advanced Practice Manager, Providence, Rhode Island

MARY G. CAREY, PhD, RN, FAAN
Director, Clinical Nursing Research Center, University of Rochester Medical Center, Rochester, New York

NANCY CASSELLA, RN, BSN, CCRN-K
Department of Medicine, Yale New Haven Hospital, New Haven, Connecticut

LAURA A. DE VAUX, MSN, RN, CNL
Department of Medicine, Yale New Haven Hospital, New Haven, Connecticut

JUSTIN DILIBERO, DNP, APRN, CCRN-K, CCNS, ACCNS-AG, FCNS
Chair, Graduate Department, Director, Doctor of Nursing Practice Program, Assistant Professor, Rhode Island College School of Nursing, Rhode Island Nurse Education Center, Providence, Rhode Island

MELISSA GORMAN, MSN, RN, NPD-BC, CCRN-K
Education Coordinator, Shriners Hospitals for Children-Boston, Boston, Massachusetts

NICOLE KUPCHIK, MN, RN, CCNS, CCRN-K, PCCN-K
CEO & Clinical Nurse Specialist, Nicole Kupchik Consulting, Inc, Clinical Nurse Specialist, Evergreen Health, Seattle, Washington

DAVID LENT, DNP, MS, RN, CNL, CCRN-K, PCCN-K
Senior Clinical Nurse Leader, Adult Critical Care Outcomes, University of Rochester Medical Center, Rochester, New York

KARA MISTO, PhD, RN
Director for Professional Practice and Innovation, Rhode Island Hospital, Providence, Rhode Island

JODI E. MULLEN, MS, RN-BC, CCRN, CCNS, ACCNS-P, FCCM
Clinical Leader, Pediatric Intensive Care Unit, UF Health Shands Children's Hospital, Gainesville, Florida

KEVIN SIGOVITCH, MSN, RN, NE-BC
Department of Medicine, Yale New Haven Hospital, New Haven, Connecticut

EMILY KATHERINE VALCIN, DNP, RN, CNL, CCRN-K
Director, Adult Critical Care Nursing, University of Rochester Medical Center, Rochester, New York

MACKENZIE WHITE, MS, RN
Clinical Nurse Specialist, Burn/Trauma ICU, Adult Critical Care, University of Rochester Medical Center, Rochester, New York

FIONA A. WINTERBOTTOM, DNP, MSN, APRN, ACNS-BC, ACHPN, CCRN
Clinical Nurse Specialist, Critical Care Medicine, Ochsner Health, Pulmonary Critical Care, Ochsner Medical Center, New Orleans, Louisiana

Contents

> Shock from all causes carries a high mortality. Rapid and intentional intervention to resuscitate can reduce mortality and organ injury. Approaches to fluid resuscitation, vasopressor use as well as commonly assessed laboratory values are reviewed in this paper.

> Trauma is a leading cause of death. Optimal outcomes depend on a coordinated effort. Providers must be prepared to act in an organized and methodical manner. Recognizing and immediately treating causes of shock after trauma offer the best chance of survival to the patient. Incorporating evidence-based knowledge and resuscitation techniques learned from the military, the trauma victim experiencing acute hypovolemia has better outcomes because of advances in the clinical management of blood loss than ever before. Treatment focuses primarily on stopping the bleeding, providing damage control resuscitation, and monitoring and treating the patient for signs of shock. If the patient can be stabilized and avoid the lethal trauma triad, definitive surgical care can be achieved.

> Sepsis is recognized as a major health care problem worldwide. In the United States, mortality from severe sepsis and septic shock remains a serious health problem; yet, the early recognition of sepsis by nurses reduces can reduce mortality, morbidity, and long-term consequences of sepsis for patients. Improving the knowledge of nurses to first recognize the early signs of sepsis and then how to apply the most up-to-date evidence-based treatments can improve outcomes. Enhanced monitoring includes the use of computerized early warning systems to alert nurses of worrisome clinical patterns and promote the early recognition of sepsis.

> Serious burn injuries may have lifelong impacts for individuals that experience them and require timely medical treatment in order to reduce associated morbidity and mortality. Initial management of a burn is nursing intensive and focuses primarily on stopping the burning process, maintaining homeostasis by keeping the patient warm, and replacing lost fluid and

electrolytes. As healing progresses, nurses meet the critical needs of the patient and must skillfully manage pain levels, perform burn care, prevent infection, help the patient meet increased nutrient requirements, and address psychological concerns with the goal to restore health and function to the highest possible level.

This article describes evidence-based nursing practices for detecting pediatric decompensation and prevention of cardiopulmonary arrest and outlines the process for effective and high-quality pediatric resuscitation and postresuscitation care. Primary concepts include pediatric decompensation signs and symptoms, pediatric resuscitation essential practices, and postresuscitation care, monitoring, and outcomes. Pediatric-specific considerations for family presence during resuscitation, ensuring good outcomes for medically complex children in community settings, and the role of targeted temperature management, continuous electroencephalography, and the use of extracorporeal membrane oxygenation in pediatric resuscitation are also discussed.

And that reference citations are not used in the synopsis. A devastating complication of cardiac arrest is hypoxic-ischemic injury, which leads to neurologic dysfunction and subsequently high mortality. Post–cardiac arrest care is complex and requires a multimodal approach to manage hemodynamic instability as well as provide neuroprotection. Targeted temperature management is recommended by the American Heart Association as well as the International Liaison Committee on Resuscitation as a class 1 intervention for postarrest neuroprotection in patients who remain unresponsive after cardiac arrest.

Patients who experience an in-hospital cardiopulmonary arrest event often have poor outcomes. Those outcomes are influenced by institutional factors, including the effectiveness of the responding team. Two main types of response teams may exist for in-hospital settings: basic life support trained staff providing initial interventions, and advanced cardiac life support teams. The interface between these two responses, and differences in discipline, experience, and skill mix, adds complexity to team dynamics. In-hospital cardiopulmonary arrest teams benefit from addressing these and other factors, which may lead to lack of clarity in role and responsibility identification and ultimately team performance.

Family presence during cardiopulmonary resuscitation (FPDR) is an evidence-based practice in the hospital setting. Members of the interdisciplinary team should adhere to ethical principles and patient and family-centered care concepts when offering interventions to support the family member during this potential end-of-life crisis. FPDR is an option for family members who are interested, screened as appropriate, and supported by a family facilitator. Essential components to guide this practice include developing an FPDR policy, educating the health care team, and creating evaluation methods.

Cardiac arrest is a significant cause of morbidity and mortality in the United States. Cardiac arrest can occur in the community or among hospitalized patients. There are many commonalities between in-hospital cardiac arrest (IHCA) and out-of-hospital cardiac arrest; however, significant differences exist. Optimizing outcomes for patients with IHCA depends on high-quality care supported by the best available evidence. It is essential that critical care nurses are familiar with the evidence related to IHCA. This article focuses on a review of the evidence on IHCA, focusing on practical implications for critical care nursing practice.

Tele-critical care (TCC) is a health care delivery model that connects medical information, interprofessional teams, patients, and families through advanced pathways, such as audio-video interfaces, machine learning, risk prediction algorithms, smart alarms, artificial intelligence, and physiologic sensing devices. TCC expands critical care services and expertise beyond the walls of the intensive care unit to logistic centers, emergency departments, general wards, war zones, disaster settings, and pandemics. This article describes the broad use of TCC for rescue and resuscitation and provides case presentations.

CRITICAL CARE NURSING
CLINICS OF NORTH AMERICA

SERIES OF RELATED INTEREST

Nursing Clinics of North America http://www.nursing.theclinics.com
Advances in Family Practice Nursing www.advancesinfamilypracticenursing.com

THE CLINICS ARE AVAILABLE ONLINE!
Access your subscription at:
www.theclinics.com

Preface

Resuscitation in Critical Care

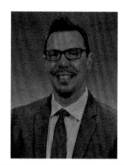

Justin DiLibero, DNP, APRN, CCRN-K, CCNS, ACCNS-AG, FCNS
Editor

Resuscitate means to revive from apparent death or from unconsciousness.[1] While the term resuscitation often brings to mind a patient in cardiac arrest receiving CPR, the concept is much broader in scope. At the most basic level, resuscitation refers to the restoration and maintenance of perfusion at the cellular and tissue levels. This is a hallmark of critical care.

Critical care is a specialized area of nursing and medicine focused on the treatment of patients with actual or impending life-threatening illness or injury that, without treatment, will result in death. Critical care focuses on the provision of resuscitation and supportive care, while the underlying process is reversed. Although historically limited to the intensive care unit (ICU), critically ill patients are increasingly cared for in other areas of the hospital or even in the community setting. From this perspective, critical care is most appropriately defined as the provision of "rapid resuscitative and supportive care where it is needed...."[2]

The first ICU can be traced back to1854 during the Crimean War, where Florence Nightingale moved the most seriously injured soldiers near the nurses' station so they could be more closely monitored.[2,3] The modern ICU began with the development of the mechanical ventilator used to support polio patients in the 1950s.[2,3] Since the inception of critical care, advances in science and technology have transformed practice. In the past, critically ill patients received invasive monitoring, deep sedation, and highly restricted visitation.[3] Today, the focus is on increasingly less-invasive or noninvasive monitoring, conservative sedation, open visitation, and more patient- and family-centered approaches to care.[3]

Advances in science and technology related to resuscitation are evolving rapidly. New evidence supports a more complete understanding of the pathophysiology of critical illnesses. Updated guidelines support consistent, evidence-based approaches to the care of specific patient populations, such as those with sepsis, cardiac arrest,

Crit Care Nurs Clin N Am 33 (2021) ix–x
https://doi.org/10.1016/j.cnc.2021.06.001
0899-5885/21/© 2021 Published by Elsevier Inc.

trauma, and burns. Scientific advances also support the development of innovative systems and processes of care. For example, tele-critical care units are expanding the availability of critical care support both within and outside of ICUs, and formal resuscitation teams are facilitating earlier identification of at-risk patients and standardizing the delivery of best practices at the bedside.

As members of a multidisciplinary team, critical care nurses play an essential role in delivering the best evidence-based practices throughout the phases of resuscitation. As the provider with the closest proximity to the bedside, critical care nurses perform the majority of patient assessments and are generally the first to identify the often-subtle signs of clinical deterioration. Critical care nurses are typically the first to initiate life-sustaining therapies and apply the art and science of nursing to the assessment, planning, intervention, and evaluation of patients through all phases of care from admission through discharge. Although many things have changed over the years, one thing has not: the quality of nursing care remains one of the most important predictors of patient outcomes. The ability to provide the highest quality of nursing care depends on the nurse's knowledge and skill in applying the best available evidence to practice.

This issue of *Critical Care Nursing Clinics of North America* covers the most recent evidence across a broad range of topics related to resuscitation. Articles have been contributed by authors who are experts in their area of practice. We hope this issue will support critical care nurses in the delivery of the best evidence-based practices that will ultimately contribute to optimal patient outcomes.

Justin DiLibero, DNP, APRN, CCRN-K, CCNS, ACCNS-AG, FCNS
Rhode Island College
350 Eddy Street
Providence, RI 02903, USA

E-mail address:
jdilibero@ric.edu

REFERENCES

1. Miriam-Webster. Incorporated. Miriam-Webster. 2021. Available at: https://www.merriam-webster.com/dictionary/resuscitate. Accessed March 30, 2021.
2. Marshall J, Bosco L, Adhikari N, et al. What is an intensive care unit? A report from the task force of the World Federation of Societies of Intensive and Critical Medicine. J Crit Care 2021;37:270–6.
3. Vincent J. Critical care—where have we been and where are we going? Crit Care 2013;17:1–6.

Principles of Resuscitation

Nicole Kupchik, MN, RN, CCNS, CCRN-K, PCCN-K*

KEYWORDS

- Fluid resuscitation • Fluid overload • Fluid responsiveness • Passive leg raise test
- Stroke volume • Lactate • Lactate clearance • Resuscitation endpoints

KEY POINTS

- Overresuscitation or underresuscitation in shock states can lead to poor outcomes.
- Fluid overload can cause complications, resulting in edema, lung injury, intraabdominal hypertension, immobility, and increased hospital length of stay.
- When the passive leg raise test is combined with a stroke volume measure to guide fluid resuscitation, it leads to less fluid administered, less mechanical ventilation, less renal replacement therapy, and decreased intensive care unit and hospital length of stay.
- The type of fluid used to resuscitate patients matters. Hyperchloremia from excessive saline administration may lead to kidney injury.
- Lactate is a commonly assessed laboratory value used as a surrogate marker of tissue perfusion and oxygenation; however, it has limitations.
- Lactate clearance is helpful in prognostication in shock states.

SHOCK

Shock from any cause is life-threatening and carries high mortality. It has been recently described as circulatory failure that leads to inadequate cellular oxygen utilization.[1] Shock leads to a vicious cycle of tissue and cellular hypoxia with oxygen consumption and delivery imbalances. In various states of shock, it is important to understand what is happening from a hemodynamic standpoint. **Table 1** provides a summary of expected hemodynamic changes in different shock states.

Anticipating expected hemodynamic alterations such as cardiac output (CO), preload, and afterload will aid in clinical decision-making. A study conducted in 2010 identified septic shock as being the most common type of shock, followed by cardiogenic and then hypovolemic shock.[2] The goal in treating patients with shock is to support adequate perfusion through resuscitation measures while reversing underlying causes.

CEO & Clinical Nurse Specialist, Nicole Kupchik Consulting, Inc., P.O. Box 28053, WA, 98188, USA; Clinical Nurse Specialist, Evergreen Health, P.O. Box 28053, WA 98188, USA
* Corresponding author.
E-mail address: info@kupchikconsulting.com

Crit Care Nurs Clin N Am 33 (2021) 225–244
https://doi.org/10.1016/j.cnc.2021.05.001
0899-5885/21/© 2021 Elsevier Inc. All rights reserved.

CASE

A 62-year-old woman presented to the emergency department with a progressive productive cough, fever, and chills. Her husband stated she was "out of it" and described her as being lethargic compared with her baseline.

Past medical history includes hypertension controlled well with a diuretic and angiotensin-converting enzyme inhibitor and hyperlipidemia treated with a daily statin medication.

Two 18-gauge peripheral intravenous catheters were inserted in her left hand and forearm. Laboratory findings were obtained, including 2 sets of blood cultures; complete blood count with differential; chemistry panel; and venous lactate, procalcitonin, and bilirubin levels. Because of hypotension with an mean arterial pressure (MAP) of 58 mm Hg, 2 L (30 mL/kg) of lactated Ringer solution was each rapidly bolused over 15 to 20 minutes. Intravenous (IV) antibiotics were started for suspected community-acquired pneumonia. Acetaminophen was also administered to treat her fever.

	Admission to the ED	1 h Later
HR (bpm)	110	102
BP (mm Hg)	80/48 (59)	88/46 (60)
RR (bpm)	32	30
EtCO$_2$ (mm Hg)	28	32
SpO$_2$	90%	92%
O$_2$ administration	Room air	4-L cannula
Temperature	38.6°C (101.5°F)	38.1°C (100.5°F)
Lactate (mmol/L)	4.2	3.8
Procalcitonin (ng/mL)	22	-

The patient continued to exhibit hypotension with an elevated lactate level despite receiving 2 L of fluid. Many of us have been in the clinical situation where we ask, does the patient need additional fluid, or should a vasopressor be initiated to treat the hypotension? If an inadequate volume of fluid is administered, it can lead to circulatory collapse. If too much fluid is administered, it can lead to edema and complications of fluid overload. If a vasopressor is considered, when should it be initiated in relationship to fluid resuscitation? Is a vasopressor is started, the patient will most likely need to be admitted to critical care, which may be a barrier due to limited resources.

BASIC PRINCIPLES OF RESUSCITATION

Resuscitation of critically ill patients will vary depending on the shock state. It is important to have solid knowledge of hemodynamic concepts, especially CO and stroke volume (SV), preload, afterload, and tissue oxygenation. At the bedside we do not always have technology readily available to provide hemodynamic profiles; however, having a baseline understanding of each will assist in guiding therapy. **Table 2** outlines hemodynamic variables used clinically. There are some general principles that apply to any resuscitation event:

- Do not cause harm by overresuscitation or underresuscitation
- Clearly establish the goals and clear end points of resuscitation for the patient (eg, lactate and lactate clearance, MAP target, SV target, etc.)
- Preserve perfusion and blood flow to limit organ injury
- Intervene to stop bleeding and correct any associated coagulopathy
- Early intervention may improve mortality and ideally minimize long-term disability

Table 1
Expected hemodynamic changes in different shock states

Type of Shock	CO/SV	Preload	Afterload	SvO_2/ $ScvO_2$	Resuscitation
Septic/ Vasogenic	↑ if hyperdynamic, ↓ later and with cardiac dysfunction	Early ↓/↑	↓	↓, late ↑	Fluid initially, then vasopressors, + inotrope
Cardiogenic	↓	↑	↑	↓	+ Inotropes, vasopressors, diuretics, mechanical assistance (Impella or IABP)
Hypovolemic	↓	↓	↑	↓	Volume expansion—fluid or blood; locate and treat bleeding if indicated
Obstructive (Tamponade)	↓	↑	↑	↓	Pericardiocentesis, reverse coagulopathy, identify bleeding if indicated

Data from Kulkarni AP, Kothekar AT & Divatia JV. Textbook of Hemodynamic Monitoring and Therapy in the Critically Ill. Jaypee Brothers Medical Publishing. P. 2019 and Marino, P. The ICU Book, 4th edition P. 2014. Section IV. Disorders of circulatory flow. Wolters Kluwer, Lippincott Williams & Wilkins. p. 193–279.

THE DETRIMENT OF FLUID IMBALANCE

The initial priority in treating shock is to assess and optimize intravascular volume. When resuscitating patients with fluid, it is important to ask the following questions: When to give fluid? Which type of fluid? How much fluid? When should we stop giving fluid?

Table 3 summarizes complications associated with imbalances of fluid in critically ill patients. In shock states, underresuscitation can lead to uncorrected tissue hypoperfusion and tissue hypoxia, acute kidney injury, splanchnic ischemia, multisystem organ dysfunction, and circulatory collapse.[3,4]

The opposite end of the spectrum is fluid overload, which is equally as dangerous and not uncommon. When patients are fluid overloaded it can lead to peripheral and organ edema, increased lung water that can progress to lung injury and acute respiratory distress syndrome (ARDS), intrabdominal hypertension and compartment syndrome, acute kidney injury, delirium, organ failure, increased ventilator days, as well as increased intensive care unit (ICU) and hospital length of stay and higher mortality.[5–9]

Marik and colleagues (2017) evaluated a large database of patients with severe sepsis and septic shock, identifying statistically and clinically significant complications when large volumes of fluid were administered during the first day of admission. Fluid overload was an independent predictor of mortality and associated with nonreversible patient risks including renal dysfunction and pulmonary complications. When 5 to greater than 9 L of fluid was administered on the first day of hospital admission,

Table 2
Hemodynamic variables

Hemodynamic Variable	Definition	How to Estimate It
Preload	The stretch of the myocardium at the end of diastole	Right ventricle: Central venous pressure (CVP) Right ventricular end-diastolic volume (RVEDV) Left ventricle: Pulmonary artery occlusive pressure (PAOP) Left ventricular end-diastolic volume (LVEDV)
Afterload	The resistance the ventricles must overcome to eject its blood volume	Pulmonary vascular resistance (PVR)—right ventricular afterload Systemic vascular resistance (SVR)—left ventricular afterload
Contractility	The shortening of the myocardial muscle; the innate ability of the myocardium to contract	Left ventricular ejection fraction (LVEF)
Stroke volume (SV)	The amount of blood ejected from the ventricles with each heart beat; influenced by preload, afterload, and contractility	End diastolic volume (EDV)–end systolic volume (ESV)
Cardiac output (CO)	The amount of blood ejected from the ventricles per minute—liters per minute	Heart rate x stroke volume
Mixed venous oxygenation	The measurement of saturated oxygen in the blood before it is transported to the lungs	$SvO_2/ScvO_2$

Data from Refs[60–62]

Table 3
The complications of fluid imbalance

Fluid Resuscitation Complications		
Too Much Fluid	**Optimal Fluid**	**Not Enough Fluid**
Tissue edema Organ edema Mechanical ventilation Kidney injury ARDS Intraabdominal hypertension Death		Refractory hypotension Tissue hypoperfusion Organ failure Circulatory collapse Death

Data from Refs[3–7]

mortality increased by 2.3% for each additional liter greater than 5 L ($P = .0003$), and the total hospital cost increased by almost $1000 for each liter greater than 5 L ($P = .005$).[9]

The long-term effects of fluid overload can lead to significant adverse consequences. Mitchell and colleagues conducted a retrospective analysis to determine outcomes related to fluid overload among 247 patients with septic shock.[10] In this study, volume overload was defined as an increase of 10% of admission body weight at ICU discharge to an acute care unit. Eighty-six percent of patients had a positive fluid balance and 35% experienced volume overload at ICU discharge. Patients averaged 12.5 L positive fluid balance with a median of 5.2 L; however, only 42% received diuretics during hospitalization. In this study, volume overload was associated with an inability to ambulate at discharge. In addition, a greater percentage of patients who were volume overloaded were discharged to a health care facility versus home.

Malbrain and colleagues described the 4 phases of fluid resuscitation (**Table 4**). The 4 phases need to be considered in the patient's overall cumulative fluid balance. The initial phase is the "rescue phase"—the first minutes to hours a patient presents with hypotension. We then move to the "optimization phase," where we cease fluid administration if the patient is no longer fluid responsive and move to other therapies if hypotension ensues. The "stabilization phase" can last days with the goal of hemodynamic stability while optimizing tissue perfusion. Finally, the "evacuation phase" can take days to weeks with the goal of returning the patient to their baseline.[11,12]

Unfortunately, during the rescue and optimization phases, fluid is often administered without appropriately assessing if the patient is fluid responsive. Fluids should be considered a drug. They need to be dosed appropriately based on appropriate physiologic response to fluid challenges. One may argue that the fourth phase of evacuation and using diuretics to correct fluid overload is an older paradigm and outdated approach to fluid management. Perhaps the goal should be focused on avoiding fluid overload by administering resuscitation fluid only if the patient if hypoperfused and fluid responsive.

Back to the initial question—how do I know if my hypotensive patient needs additional fluid or if a vasopressor should be started? The answer is, if additional fluid is administered, the expected response should demonstrate an increase in SV. This hemodynamic concept known as the Frank-Starling curve represents the relationship between ventricular preload and SV. When a patient is no longer fluid responsive, other therapies such as vasopressors or positive inotropes should be explored to treat hypoperfusion.

Table 4		
The four phases of fluid resuscitation for shock		
Phase	**Timing**	**Goal**
Resuscitation	First 3–6 h of presentation	Hemodynamic stability: initial rapid fluid boluses for hypotension, then consider fluid responsiveness techniques
Optimization	Hours following	Organ and tissue perfusion, hemodynamic stability
Stabilization	Days following	Minimize damage if fluid overloaded, more tailored therapy to support hemodynamics if needed
Evacuation	Days to weeks	Fluid removal, negative fluid balance

Adapted from Malbrain MLNG, Van Regenmortel N, Saugel B, et al. Principles of fluid management and stewardship in septic shock: it is time to consider the four D's and the four phases of fluid therapy. Ann Intensive Care. 2018;8(1):66; with permission.

DO HEART RATE AND BLOOD PRESSURE ACCURATELY PREDICT FLUID RESPONSIVENESS?

The answer is no. Blood pressure is affected by both arterial tone and intravascular volume. Arterial vasoconstriction can normalize blood pressure and hide hypovolemia. The arterial response to intravenous volume expansion is unpredictable. If fluid administration is aimed to restore and maintain arterial blood pressure, it can lead to unnecessary fluid overload, delayed vasoactive therapy, and increased mortality. Blood pressure is a late sign of hypovolemia. In a study of healthy volunteers, noninvasive blood pressure did not predict fluid responders when compared with the passive leg raise (PLR) test used with a noninvasive SV measurement.[13]

CAN CENTRAL VENOUS PRESSURE BE USED TO GUIDE FLUID ADMINISTRATION?

The practice of using central venous pressure as a target for fluid administration has been questioned and largely abandoned.[14–16] A systematic review published in 2008 demonstrated central venous pressure is a static hemodynamic variable and poor indicator of volume status and changes in CVP do not predict fluid responsiveness. In addition, CVP values are affected by positive pressure mechanical ventilation, positive end-expiratory pressure, and any cause of increased intrathoracic pressure. CVP may be an acceptable indicator of right ventricular preload but not fluid responsiveness.[17]

When compared with other hemodynamic parameters such as SV changes, the area under the curve (AUC) of the CVP to predict fluid responsiveness is 0.56[18]; this equates to the predictability of the CVP to determine fluid responsiveness is as accurate as the flip of a coin—about a 50/50 chance. Clinically, any technology or therapy scoring an AUC less than 0.7 should not be used to make clinical decisions, as the margin of error is too large.

Historically, shock treatment guidelines recommended using CVP to guide fluid resuscitation, often targeting a CVP of at least 8 to 12 mm Hg and higher if the patient was receiving mechanical ventilation.[3] Findings from the VASST trial identified the CVP to be an unreliable measure of fluid balance after 12 hours of initial resuscitation.[6] The Surviving Sepsis Campaign Guidelines recommend if shock is not resolving, use a dynamic over static variable such as CVP to guide/predict fluid responsiveness.[19] The bottom line is that based on the literature, CVP should not be used to guide fluid resuscitation.

Has there been a change in practice over time? **Table 5** compares 3 studies published over the past 10 years. Even though it does not predict fluid responsiveness, blood pressure was still the most commonly used parameter to make fluid decisions.[14–16,20] Over time, there has been a notable decrease in the use of CVP to guide fluid administration.

Dynamic measures of fluid responsiveness measure the change in SV related to an increase in preload/venous return. Two strategies used to assess fluid responsiveness with stroke volume measures include the passive leg raise (PLR) test or administration of a fluid bolus challenge. These strategies are used with technology that measures SV and CO to provide a physiologic challenge in hypotensive patients to identify the appropriate therapy.

FLUID RESPONSIVENESS

If the patient's SV does not increase with a physiologic or fluid challenge, then an assessment of other therapies, such as vasopressors or positive inotropes, should be explored. Fluid underresuscitation and overresuscitation is detrimental. Clinical

Table 5			
What drives administration a fluid bolus: practice change over time			
Indicator	SAFE 2004[20] (n = %)	SAFE-TRIPS 2010[14] (n = %)	Fluid-TRIPS 2014[15] (n = %)
BP	67.9	63.7	71.8
CVP	54.8	19.5	11.2
HR	59.8	52.3	30
UOP	54.8	30	41
Capillary refill	55.2	12.4	20.1

Data from Refs[14–16,20]

practices of blindly administering fluid without using a physiologic indicator should be avoided, as there are significant negative clinical consequences.

Fluid responsiveness is defined in the literature as an increase in SV of greater than or equal to 10% after the patient receives 500 mL of crystalloid over 10 to 15 minutes or a shift in fluids (physiologic bolus) by the PLR test.[21] **Table 6** outlines invasive and noninvasive hemodynamic technologies with the ability to measure or estimate fluid responsiveness with SV changes.

THE PASSIVE LEG RAISE TEST

The PLR test is a dynamic test that can positively predict fluid responsiveness when used in conjunction with an SV measure. The test is performed by passively raising the legs for 2 to 3 minutes, which then transfers blood from legs and abdominal compartment toward the heart. It is the equivalent of giving the patient a physiologic fluid challenge without administering fluid. **Fig. 1** highlights the directions to perform this test.

To perform the PLR test, a baseline SV measure is obtained with the patient in the supine position and the head of bed elevated 45°. Once the baseline SV is established, the head is quickly lowered to the flat position and the legs passively raised to 45°. The SV is then reevaluated after 2 to 3 minutes. In the setting of hypotension, if the SV increases by greater than or equal to 10%, this indicates the patient is likely fluid responsive. If the SV does not increase by at least 10%, the patient is unlikely fluid responsive and the hypotension should be treated with a vasopressor. In the setting of cardiac dysfunction, the patient should be evaluated for the need of a positive inotrope such as dobutamine.

Limitations to the PLR test include intraabdominal hypertension, head trauma or intracranial pressure issues, lower extremity deep vein thrombosis, severe

Table 6	
Hemodynamic technology options to measure cardiac output and stroke volume	
Noninvasive Technologies	**Invasive Technologies**
Bioreactance	Arterial line technologies (including PPV, SVV)
Digit continuous CO devices	Esophageal Doppler
Ultrasound CO measurement (USCOM)	Pulmonary artery catheter (measures right ventricular CO and SV)
Ultrasound (used to estimate inferior vena cava collapse)	Note: the PA catheter should not be used with the PLR test, as CO and SV averaging is delayed

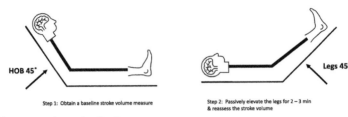

Step 1: Obtain a baseline stroke volume measure

Step 2: Passively elevate the legs for 2 – 3 min & reassess the stroke volume

Fig. 1. The passive leg raise (PLR) test.

hypovolemia and/or hemorrhage, and lower extremity amputations. In addition, venous compression stockings should be removed before performing the PLR test. If a patient has contraindications to the PLR test, a 250 to 500 mL fluid bolus may be rapidly administered in conjunction with preinfusion and postinfusion SV measurement.

A recently published meta-analysis of the PLR test evaluated 21 studies assessing PLR with SV/CO or pulse pressure and included measurements obtained by echocardiogram, pulse contour analysis, Bioreactance, esophageal Doppler, pulmonary artery catheter, and suprasternal Doppler. When the PLR test was used with CO/SV, the ability to positively predict fluid responsiveness scored an AUC of 0.95, meaning the test is an excellent predictor. When the PLR test was used with pulse pressure change, the ability to positively predict fluid responsiveness scored an AUC of 0.77[22]; this is a fair predictor, but there will be a greater margin of error compared with an SV measure.

CLINICAL OUTCOME STUDIES

In 2017, the University of Kansas conducted a nonrandomized comparison study evaluating outcomes of patients with severe sepsis and septic shock who received usual care to guide fluid administration versus SV changes with Bioreactance/noninvasive CO measurements.[23]

Ninety-one patients were included in the usual care group and 100 patients in the group guided by SV changes using the Bioreactance device. In the usual care arm, no specific technology was used, only vital signs and lactate levels to determine fluid needs in hypotensive patients.

The arm using the Bioreactance technology measured changes in SV to identify fluid responsiveness. The Bioreactance sensors were placed on patients in the early phases of resuscitation. Interestingly, only 53% of patients needed treatment with additional fluid in the Bioreactance group; this is consistent with other studies, reinforcing there are a proportion of patients who are unlikely to improve perfusion with additional fluid.

The clinical results were favorable for those enrolled in the Bioreactance group. When SV changes were used to guide treatment, patients received:

- An average difference of 3.59 L less fluid (P = .002)
- An average of 32.78 fewer hours of vasopressor requirements (P = .001)
- Statistically significant decreased need for mechanical ventilation (P = .0001)
- Decreased length of stay in the ICU—average difference 2.89 days (P = .03)

Building on that study was a multicenter, nonblinded, randomized controlled trial (RCT) evaluating SV-guided fluid resuscitation compared with usual care in patients with refractory septic shock. The FRESH Trial enrolled 124 patients from 13 US and

UK hospitals randomized in a 2:1 enrollment; 83 patients were resuscitated using SV changes, and 41 patients received usual care.

Enrollment requirements included patients from the emergency department who received less than 3 L of fluid administration. The PLR test with dynamic measure of SV change using Bioreactance technology was used to guide the decision of fluid versus vasopressors for clinical hypoperfusion. Patients were studied over the following 72 hours of care or until ICU discharge. In the study hypoperfusion was defined as (1) MAP less than 65 mm Hg, (2) persistent hyperlactemia, or (3) cryptic shock—lactate greater than 4 mmol/L without hypotension.

The primary and secondary endpoints of the study revealed similar results to the 2017 trial:

Primary endpoint: decreased 72-hour fluid balance.

- SV-guided (treatment) group: 0.65 ± 2.85 L
- Control group: 2.02 ± 3.44 L
- Favoring treatment group: −1.37 L (P = .02)

Secondary endpoints:
Renal replacement therapy needs:

- SV-guided (treatment) group: 5.1%
- Control group: 17.5% (P = .04)

Mechanical ventilation needs:

- SV-guided (treatment) group: 17.7%
- Control group: 34.1% (P = .04)

ICU length of stay:

- SV-guided (treatment) group: 3.31 days
- Control group: 6.22 days (P = .11)

Note: although the findings were not statistically significant, a decrease in the length of stay of almost 3 days is clinically and financially significant.

Discharged to home:

- SV-guided (treatment) group: 63.9%
- Control group: 43.9% (P = .035)

Some key take home points of both trials demonstrated using SV guidance with the PLR test in patients with septic shock is safe, reduced fluid balance at 72 hours as well as the total amount of fluid administered, decreased the incidence of mechanical ventilation and renal replacement therapy, and resulted in more discharges home.[24] When comparing the University of Kansas study, the FRESH Trial, and the surgical literature, the treatment effect may be more about the timing of fluid administration and identifying when the patient can use fluid to improve SV and CO. Perhaps it is not simply about giving less fluid; additional research warranted to explore this notion.

BACK TO OUR CASE

A clinically hypoperfused and hypotensive patient has a noninvasive SV monitor placed to identify if they are fluid responsive. She has previously received 30 mL/kg of IV lactated Ringer solution. A PLR test is conducted to determine fluid responsiveness.

Example 1:

Parameter	Before Passive Leg Raise (PLR) Test	2 min After Leg Raise
HR (bpm)	102	102
BP (mm Hg)	88/46 (60)	92/42 (59)
Cardiac index (L/min/m²)	4.82	5.64
Stroke volume (ml/beat)	84	98
Stroke volume index (ml/beat/m²)	47.45	55.36
Total peripheral resistance (dynes/s/cm⁻⁵)	489	-
Lactate (mmol/L)	3.8	-

Clinical action: in this example there was a *16.6% increase in SV* with the PLR test in the setting of hypotension, which indicates the patient would likely be fluid responsive. This increase does not tell you how much fluid to administer, only that the patient will likely increase their SV in response to fluid. In addition, the total peripheral resistance value is low, indicating decreased vascular resistance and vasodilation.

Example 2:

Parameter	Before Passive Leg Raise (PLR) Test	2 min After Leg Raise
HR (bpm)	102	102
BP (mm Hg)	88/46 (60)	92/42 (59)
Cardiac index (L/min/m²)	4.82	5.02
Stroke volume (ml/beat)	84	88
Stroke volume index (ml/beat/m²)	47.45	49.71
Total peripheral resistance (dynes/s/cm⁻⁵)	489	-
Lactate (mmol/L)	3.8	-

Clinical action: in this example there was a *4.8% increase in SV* in the setting of hypotension; this indicates the patient would NOT likely be fluid responsive. In this situation a vasopressor such as norepinephrine should be initiated to treat the hypotension.

TYPE OF FLUID USED TO RESUSCITATE

For decades, 0.9% sodium chloride has been one of the most commonly used resuscitation fluids. The practice has been recently questioned and a building body of evidence is supporting a move away from saline. PlasmaLyte-A and 0.9% sodium chloride were compared for fluid resuscitation in patients with diabetic ketoacidosis (DKA) as well as a comparison of saline versus Plasma-Lyte A in the initial resuscitation of patients with trauma. Both favored the use of Plasma-Lyte A.[25,26]

Why after all these years are we questioning the use of 0.9% sodium chloride? Some of the issues hypothesized with excessive administration of 0.9% sodium chloride include the development of hyperchloremia and metabolic acidosis, which may lead to renal vasoconstriction, reduced renal blood flow and increased risk of kidney injury, need for renal replacement therapy in the ICU, and increased risk for lung injury.[27,28] In addition, excessive chloride administration has been identified as an independent risk factor for in-hospital mortality.[29,30]

Table 7 compares the differences in composition of 3 commonly used isotonic IV fluid solutions. Sodium chloride has a low pH and contains a high concentration of

Table 7
Comparison of isotonic fluid composition

	0.9% Sodium Chloride	Lactated Ringer Solution	Plasma-Lyte A
pH	5.5	6.75	7.4
Osmolality (mOsm/L)	308	273	294
Na$^+$ (mEq/L)	154	130	140
K$^+$ (mEq/L)	0	4	5
Cl$^-$ (mEq/L)	154	109	98

sodium and chloride versus lactated Ringer solution and Plasma-Lyte A. Sodium chloride may be more appropriate in the setting of hyponatremia and hypochloremia, whereas Plasma-Lyte A, which has a composition closer to serum plasma, may be a better resuscitation fluid. Each fluid is a different drug with different indications.

In 2018, 2 RCTs enrolling more than 29,000 patients compared the general administration of 0.9% sodium chloride with balanced fluids—lactated Ringer solution and Plasma-Lyte A. The SALT-ED trial enrolled 13,347 noncritically ill patients comparing saline versus balanced fluid. The study revealed an increased incidence of major adverse kidney injury events within 30 days (adjusted odd ratio 0.82; 95% confidence interval 0.70–0.95, P = .01).[31]

The SMART trial enrolled 15,802 critically ill patients comparing saline with lactated Ringer solution and Plasma-Lyte A. Approximately 33% of patients were receiving mechanical ventilation and approximately 25% were receiving vasopressor therapy. The results of this study also identified a statistically significant increased incidence of major adverse kidney injury events in those who previously received renal replacement therapy. In addition, there was a signal toward higher mortality with saline administration in the group of patients with sepsis who received saline administration.[32]

A secondary analysis of the SMART trial specifically evaluated 1641 patients who were admitted to the medical ICU with a diagnosis of sepsis.[33] This was an intriguing post hoc analysis, which demonstrated a statistically significant higher mortality, higher incidence of major adverse kidney events as well as lower rates of renal replacement therapy-free days in patients who received saline over balanced fluids. Hopefully this will spur a larger RCT evaluating the effect of resuscitation fluid choice in this patient population.

In time, our knowledge of fluid type as well as administration strategies will increase. There are a few ongoing fluid trials that may provide additional answers to outstanding clinical questions:

- PLUS trial—RCT with planned enrollment of 5000 patients evaluating mortality differences using saline versus Plasma-Lyte 148 as a resuscitation fluid in critically ill patients. The estimated enrollment completion is summer of 2021 (NCT02721654).[34,35]
- BaSICS trial—enrollment was completed in October 2020 in more than 11,000 patients evaluating balanced fluid versus 0.9% sodium chloride and at rapid bolus infusion (999 mL/h) versus slower infusion (333 mL/h) for resuscitation episodes (NCT02875873).[36,37]
- CLOVERS trial—2320 patients with sepsis comparing restrictive (vasopressors first followed by rescue fluids) versus liberal fluid therapy (fluids first followed by rescue vasopressors) on 90-day mortality. Estimated study completion is June 2021 (NCT03434028).[38,39]

VASOPRESSORS AND SHOCK

In patients who are hypotensive or hypoperfused, but not fluid responsive, vasopressor therapy is often initiated. Vasopressors cause arterial and venous vasoconstriction redistributing existing blood volume, thereby increasing blood pressure and arterial resistance. When choosing a vasopressor, it is important to understand the mechanism of action. In clinical practice, catecholamine vasopressors are primarily used as first-line agents to improve blood pressure. They work by stimulating α-1 and/or β-1 receptors. **Table 8** outlines how each vasopressor works, including noncatecholamine vasopressors.

The following are some general principles to remember with vasopressor or positive inotropic agents:

- α-1 receptor stimulation will cause generalized arterial vasoconstriction to increase blood pressure.
- β-1 receptors are located on the myocardium. Stimulation will cause the heart to beat faster and contract stronger, so you may see tachycardia with increased inotropy/CO.
- β-2 receptors are found in the lungs. Stimulation causes vasodilation and may cause hypotension.

OTHER VASOPRESSOR NOTES

The key with most therapeutics is to use them early and not as a "last ditch effort." Two other vasopressors that are commonly used as second-line vasopressors include vasopressin and angiotensin-2 (Giapreza). Both are used in distributive or vasodilatory shock states and are used in conjunction with catecholamine vasopressors.[40–42]

A small RCT of patients with trauma revealed low-dose vasopressin infusion initiated during the early phase of resuscitation decreased the number of blood products required.[43] Larger multicenter trials are needed to validate the utility of vasopressin use as a strategy to decrease blood products.

An important concept to remember is fluid responsiveness may increase after the administration of drugs with beta effect, such as norepinephrine or epinephrine. It is imperative to reassess fluid responsiveness and adjust therapy as needed in patients remaining in a hypoperfused state.

When using epinephrine as a catecholamine vasopressor or inotrope infusion, it is not uncommon to observe an elevation of serum lactate. Epinephrine likely causes an upregulation of glycolysis, generating more pyruvate than can be used by mitochondria. The excessive pyruvate is converted to lactic acid via β-2 receptors. It is likely a beneficial compensatory mechanism.[44]

LABORATORY MARKERS USED IN RESUSCITATION
Lactate

Lactate levels are commonly assessed in shock states during resuscitation and are viewed as a marker of global tissue perfusion. Lactate is not specific or predictive to a disease state but rather a marker of malperfusion.[41] In global hypoxic states, lactic acid is classically believed to be produced as a byproduct of anaerobic metabolism and used for energy. A normal lactate value is 0.5 to 1.0 mmol/L and has satisfactory agreement whether drawn from arterial or venous blood.[45–48]

Lactate is mostly cleared by the liver with a small amount cleared by the kidneys. Lactic acid normally gets converted to glucose via the Cori cycle. However, in states of hypoperfusion, lactic acid is the end product of anaerobic glycolysis. Lactate levels

Table 8
Commonly used vasopressors

	Dose Ranges	α1	β1	β2	Notes
Norepinephrine (Levophed)	5–30 mcg/min	+++	++	+	Recommended as a first-line vasopressor in sepsis
Phenylephrine (Neosynephrine)	20–200 mcg/min	++++	-	-	
Epinephrine (Adrenalin)	1–5 mcg/min	++++	++++	++	
Dopamine	1–20 mcg/kg/min	++	+++	+	Effects are dose dependent
Vasopressin	0.01–0.04 units/min	-	-	-	ADH stimulates arginine vasoreceptor (V$_1$). Risk: end-organ perfusion.
Angiotensin-2 (Giapreza)	1.25 up to 80 ng/kg/min. Maintenance no more than 40 ng/kg/min	-	-	-	Vasoconstricts; causes Na$^+$ and H$_2$0 retention through increased aldosterone release. Used in septic/distributive shock.

Data from Refs[40–42,62–64]

can increase for reasons other than hypoperfusion. It is important to remember the glycolysis pathway when troubleshooting why a patient who is not hypoperfused may exhibit hyperlactemia. **Fig. 2** outlines the process of glycolysis and reasons for elevation.

Lactate levels may be elevated for reasons other than hypoperfusion and are commonly described as type A or type B lactic acidosis (**Table 9**). When troubleshooting treatment strategies for type A lactic acidosis caused by hypoperfusion and shock (septic, cardiogenic, hypovolemic, hemorrhagic) or with causes of ischemia (ischemic bowel, necrotizing fasciitis, etc.), the focus should be on improving perfusion and the oxygen delivery/oxygen consumption mismatch. If the patient is fluid responsive, perfusion (CO and SV) may be improved by administering fluids or blood. If the patient is not fluid responsive, increasing afterload and redistributing blood flow with vasopressors will improve critical perfusion. Positive inotrope infusions such as dobutamine, milrinone, or epinephrine may be an appropriate addition for low CO states.

Correcting type B lactic acidosis, which is not caused by hypoperfusion, should be focused on identifying, then reversing or discontinuing the cause. For example, correcting thiamine deficiency will likely lower lactate levels.

In the setting of severe sepsis and septic shock, lactate levels do have some prognostic utility. Lactate levels greater than or equal to 2.5 mmol/L are associated with increased mortality. Lactate levels greater than 4 are associated with a 5-fold increase in mortality. In the state of hypoperfusion, mortality increases as lactate levels increase.[49,50] With that said there is also a shift in practice with a focus on trending lactate clearance.

Lactate value:

0 to 2.4 mmol/L 4.9% predicted mortality
2.5 to 3.9 mmol/L 9.0% predicted mortality
$\geq$ 4.0 mmol/L 28.4% predicted mortality

Lactate Clearance

Lactate clearance is often used as a surrogate for the duration and severity of global tissue hypoxia and hypoperfusion. It is used both as a diagnostic and prognostic indicator. Sustained hyperlactemia for more than 6 hours predicts increased mortality.[51] Early lactate clearance is associated with improvement in organ dysfunction and outcomes in severe sepsis and septic shock.[50,52] Higher 30-day mortality and a greater need for vasopressors were observed with lower lactate clearance in the first 24 to 48 hours of resuscitation in patients with severe sepsis and septic shock.[53]

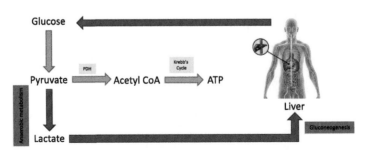

PDH = pyruvate dehydrogenase

Fig. 2. The glycolysis pathway and lactate elevation.

Table 9	
Causes of type A and type B lactic acidosis	
Type A Lactic Acidosis Causes:	**Type B Lactic Acidosis Causes:**
Shock	Renal or hepatic dysfunction
Cardiac arrest	Increased production of lactic acid and/or decreased
Hypoperfusion	clearance
Global hypoxia	Thiamine deficiency
Limb or mesenteric ischemia	Diabetic ketoacidosis (DKA)
Seizures	Alcoholism
DO_2 and Vo_2 mismatch	Medications—albuterol, epinephrine, metformin,
Anaerobic glycolysis	HIV meds

Insertion of a central line and continuous monitoring of CVP and central venous oxygen saturation ($ScvO_2$) were key elements of the early goal directed therapy protocols widely used throughout the 2000s.[3] However, when the strategy of normalizing lactate and lactate clearance was compared with normalizing $ScvO_2$ and mean arterial pressure, there was no in-hospital mortality difference.[54,55]

A recently published study of 100 patients evaluated the correlation of lactate in predicting hospital mortality. Samples were collected at baseline and after 6 hours of resuscitation. The combination of an arterial lactate greater than 3.2 mmol/L and arterial lactate clearance less than 20% was the highest predictor of mortality.[45] The Surviving Sepsis Campaign Guidelines recommend guiding resuscitation to normalize lactate in patients with elevated lactate levels as a marker of tissue hypoperfusion.[19] Caution needs to be instituted so patients are not overtreated with excessive fluid just to normalize a number. It is important to consider the big picture including lactate clearance, physical assessment, mentation, urine output, skin temperature, and presence mottling, as well as hemodynamic stability.

Arterial Base Deficit

Arterial base deficit is a marker of hypoperfusion and acidosis. It is defined as the amount of base that must be added to a liter of blood to increase the pH to 7.4, $PaCO_2$ to 40 mm Hg, and temperature to 37°C and is superior to pH as a measure of metabolic acidosis.[56] It was historically measured in severe trauma injuries and used as an adjunct endpoint of resuscitation. In general, the higher the blood loss, the greater the base deficit.[56,57] Much of the literature on base deficit was published from the 1970s to 1990s.

A normal base deficit level is less than or equal to 2 mmol/L and is commonly reported on arterial blood gas results.

Based on data from more than 16,000 patients with trauma, Mutschler and colleagues[58] redefined the severity of hypoperfusion and acidosis based on base deficit levels:

>2 to 6 mmol/L = Class II
>6 to 10 mmol/L = Class III
≥10 mmol/L = Class IV

It is important to remember base deficit values are influenced by renal failure, DKA, hyperchloremia (especially with saline administration), and chronic CO_2 retention. More recent literature points to serial lactate being superior to base deficit for predicting outcomes in critically ill.[59] If base deficit is used, it should be evaluated in conjunction with lactate and lactate clearance as well as the patient's overall hemodynamic status.

SUMMARY

Resuscitation from shock is complicated, but the guiding principle is simple. The main goal of resuscitation is restoration of tissue perfusion and oxygenation. Endpoints of resuscitation should be clearly identified and communicated with the team involved in the patient's care. Today we have better insights to understand perfusion and recognize blood pressure alone has major limitations.

With fluid resuscitation it is important to consider the type of fluid given, as well as the timing of administration. We have better tools to assess fluid responsiveness to deliver the appropriate therapy leading to improved outcomes for patients. Fluid overload has significant long-term sequelae. Recent research supports the use of dynamic hemodynamic technology to measure SV changes to guide fluid resuscitation. Additional tools such as monitoring lactate clearance can also be helpful in guiding resuscitation and predicting outcomes.

CLINICS CARE POINTS

- Signs of clinical deterioration and shock need to be recognized early.
- There is a move away from saline as a resuscitation fluid and move toward balanced fluid.
- Stroke volume guidance with the PLR test can avoid over-resuscitation which leads to numerous clinical complications.
- Lactate and lactate clearance can be helpful in resuscitation, although lactate itself has limitations.

DISCLOSURE

Speaker's Bureau: Stryker Medical & Baxter Healthcare
    Consultant: Baxter Healthcare

REFERENCES

1. Sakr Y, Reinhart K, Vincent JL, et al. Does dopamine administration in shock influence outcome? Results of the sepsis occurrence in acutely ill patients (SOAP) study. Crit Care Med 2006;34:589–97.
2. De Backer D, Biston P, Devriendt J, et al. Comparison of dopamine and norepinephrine in the treatment of shock. N Engl J Med 2010;362:779–89.
3. Rivers E, Nguyen B, Havstad S, et al, Early Goal-Directed Therapy Collaborative Group. Early goal-directed therapy in the treatment of severe sepsis and septic shock. N Engl J Med 2001;345(19):1368–77.
4. Vermeulen H, Hofland J, Legemate DA, et al. Intravenous fluid restriction after major abdominal surgery: a randomized blinded clinical trial. Trials 2009; 7(10):50.
5. Vincent JL, Sakr Y, Sprung CL, et al, Sepsis Occurrence in Acutely Ill Patients Investigators. Sepsis in European intensive care units: results of the SOAP study. Crit Care Med 2006;34(2):344–53.
6. Boyd JH, Forbes J, Nakada TA, et al. Fluid resuscitation in septic shock: a positive fluid balance and elevated central venous pressure are associated with increased mortality. Crit Care Med 2011;39(2):259–65.

7. Kelm DJ, Perrin JT, Cartin-Ceba R, et al. Fluid overload in patients with severe sepsis and septic shock treated with early goal-directed therapy is associated with increased acute need for fluid-related medical interventions and hospital death. Shock 2015;43(1):68–73.
8. Vincent JL. Fluid management in the critically ill. Kidney Int 2019;96(1):52–7.
9. Marik PE, Linde-Zwirble WT, Bittner EA, et al. Fluid administration in severe sepsis and septic shock, patterns and outcomes: an analysis of a large national database. Intensive Care Med 2017;43(5):625–32.
10. Mitchell KH, Carlbom D, Caldwell E, et al. Volume overload: prevalence, risk factors, and functional outcome in survivors of septic shock. Ann Am Thorac Soc 2015;12:1837–44.
11. Malbrain ML, Marik PE, Witters I, et al. Fluid overload, de-resuscitation, and outcomes in critically ill or injured patients: a systematic review with suggestions for clinical practice. Anaesthesiol Intensive Ther 2014;46(5):361–80.
12. Malbrain MLNG, Van Regenmortel N, Saugel B, et al. Principles of fluid management and stewardship in septic shock: it is time to consider the four D's and the four phases of fluid therapy. Ann Intensive Care 2018;8(1):66.
13. Pickett JD, Bridges E, Kritek PA, et al. Noninvasive blood pressure monitoring and prediction of fluid responsiveness to passive leg raising. Am J Crit Care 2018;27(3):228–37.
14. Finfer S, Liu B, Taylor C, et al. Resuscitation fluid use in critically ill adults: an international cross-sectional study in 391 intensive care units. Crit Care 2010;14: R185.
15. Hammond NE, Taylor C, Finfer S, et al, Fluid-TRIPS and Fluids Investigators; George Institute for Global Health, The ANZICS Clinical Trials Group, BRICNet, and the REVA research Network. Patterns of intravenous fluid resuscitation use in adult intensive care patients between 2007 and 2014: an international cross-sectional study. PLoS One 2017;12:e0176292.
16. Bihari S, Prakash S, Barnes M, et al. Why is a fluid bolus administered and has there been a change in practice? Results from SAFE, SAFE TRIPS and fluid TRIPS datasets. Intensive Care Med 2020;46(6):1284–5.
17. Marik PE, Baram M, Vahid B. Does central venous pressure predict fluid responsiveness? A systematic review of the literature and the tale of seven mares. Chest 2008;134(1):172–8.
18. Michard F, Boussat S, Chemla D, et al. Relation between respiratory changes in arterial pulse pressure and fluid responsiveness in septic patients with acute circulatory failure. Am J Respir Crit Care Med 2000;162(1):134–8.
19. Rhodes A, Evans LE, Alhazzani W, et al. Surviving sepsis campaign: international guidelines for management of sepsis and septic shock: 2016. Crit Care Med 2017;45(3):486–552.
20. Finfer S, Bellomo R, Boyce N, et al. A comparison of albumin and saline for fluid resuscitation in the intensive care unit. N Engl J Med 2004;350:2247–56.
21. Marik PE, Weinmann M. Optimizing fluid therapy in shock. Curr Opin Crit Care 2019;25(3):246–51.
22. Monnet X, Marik P, Teboul JL. Passive leg raising for predicting fluid responsiveness: a systematic review and meta-analysis. Intensive Care Med 2016;42(12): 1935–47.
23. Latham HE, Bengtson CD, Satterwhite L, et al. Stroke volume guided resuscitation in severe sepsis and septic shock improves outcomes. J Crit Care 2017; 42:42–6.

24. Douglas IS, Alapat PM, Corl KA, et al. Fluid response evaluation in sepsis hypotension and shock: a randomized clinical trial. Chest 2020;158(4):1431–45.
25. Chua HR, Venkatesh B, Stachowski E, et al. Plasma-Lyte 148 vs 0.9% saline for fluid resuscitation in diabetic ketoacidosis. J Crit Care 2012;27(2):138–45.
26. Young JB, Utter GH, Schermer CR, et al. Saline versus Plasma-Lyte A in initial resuscitation of trauma patients: a randomized trial. Ann Surg 2014;259(2): 255–62.
27. Yunos NM, Kim IB, Bellomo R, et al. The biochemical effects of restricting chloride-rich fluids in intensive care. Crit Care Med 2011;39:2419–24.
28. Yunos NM, Bellomo R, Hegarty C, et al. Association between a chloride-liberal vs chloride-restrictive intravenous fluid administration strategy and kidney injury in critically ill adults. JAMA 2012;308:1566–72.
29. Neyra JA, Canepa-Escaro F, Li X, et al, Acute Kidney Injury in Critical Illness Study Group. Association of hyperchloremia with hospital mortality in critically ill septic patients. Crit Care Med 2015;43(9):1938–44.
30. Haller JT, Smetana K, Erdman MJ, et al. An association between hyperchloremia and acute kidney injury in patients with acute ischemic stroke. Neurohospitalist 2020;10(4):250–6.
31. Self WH, Semler MW, Wanderer JP, et al, SALT-ED Investigators. Balanced crystalloids versus saline in noncritically ill adults. N Engl J Med 2018;378(9):819–28.
32. Semler MW, Wanderer JP, Ehrenfeld JM, et al, SALT Investigators and the Pragmatic Critical Care Research Group; SALT Investigators. Balanced crystalloids versus saline in the intensive care unit. the salt randomized trial. Am J Respir Crit Care Med 2017;195(10):1362–72.
33. Brown RM, Wang L, Coston TD, et al. Balanced crystalloids versus saline in sepsis. A secondary analysis of the SMART clinical trial. Am J Respir Crit Care Med 2019;200(12):1487–95.
34. Hammond NE, Bellomo R, Gallagher M, et al. The Plasma-Lyte 148 v Saline (PLUS) study protocol: a multicentre, randomised controlled trial of the effect of intensive care fluid therapy on mortality. Crit Care Resusc 2017;19:239–46.
35. Available at: https://clinicaltrials.gov/ct2/show/NCT02721654. Accessed February 21, 2021.
36. Zampieri FG, Azevedo LCP, Correa TD, et al, BaSICS Investigators and the BRIC-Net. Study protocol for the balanced solution versus saline in intensive care study (BaSICS): a factorial randomised trial. Crit Care Resusc 2017;19:175–82.
37. Available at: https://clinicaltrials.gov/ct2/show/NCT02875873. Accessed February 21, 2021.
38. Available at: https://clinicaltrials.gov/ct2/show/NCT03434028. Accessed February 21, 2021.
39. Available at: https://petalnet.org/studies/public/clovers. Accessed February 21, 2021.
40. Russell JA, Walley KR, Singer J, et al. VASST Investigators. Vasopressin versus norepinephrine infusion in patients with septic shock. N Engl J Med 2008; 358(9):877–87.
41. Gordon AC, Mason AJ, Thirunavukkarasu N, et al, VANISH Investigators. Effect of early vasopressin vs norepinephrine on kidney failure in patients with septic shock: the VANISH randomized clinical trial. JAMA 2016;316(5):509–18.
42. Khanna A, English SW, Wang XS, et al, ATHOS-3 Investigators. Angiotensin II for the treatment of vasodilatory shock. N Engl J Med 2017;377(5):419–30.
43. Sims CA, Holena D, Kim P, et al. Effect of low-dose supplementation of arginine vasopressin on need for blood product transfusions in patients with trauma and

hemorrhagic shock: a randomized clinical trial. JAMA Surg 2019;154(11): 994–1003.

44. Levy B, Perez P, Perny J, et al. Comparison of norepinephrine-dobutamine to epinephrine for hemodynamics, lactate metabolism, and organ function variables in cardiogenic shock: a prospective, randomized pilot study. Crit Care Med 2011;39(3):450-5.

45. Karon BS, Tolan NV, Wockenfus AM, et al. Evaluation of lactate, white blood cell count, neutrophil count, procalcitonin and immature granulocyte count as biomarkers for sepsis in emergency department patients. Clin Biochem 2017; 50(16–17):956–8.

46. Mahmoodpoor A, Shadvar K, Sanaie S, et al. Arterial vs venous lactate: correlation and predictive value of mortality of patients with sepsis during early resuscitation phase. J Crit Care 2020;58:118–24.

47. Younger JG, Falk JL, Rothrock SG. Relationship between arterial and peripheral venous lactate levels. Acad Emerg Med 1996;3(7):730–4.

48. Lavery RF, Livingston DH, Tortella BJ, et al. The utility of venous lactate to triage injured patients in the trauma center. J Am Coll Surg 2000;190(6):656–64.

49. Middleton P, Kelly AM, Brown J, et al. Agreement between arterial and central venous values for pH, bicarbonate, base excess, and lactate. Emerg Med J 2006;23(8):622–4.

50. Shapiro NI, Howell MD, Talmor D, et al. Serum lactate as a predictor of mortality in emergency department patients with infection. Ann Emerg Med 2005;45(5): 524–8.

51. Nguyen HB, Rivers EP, Knoblich BP, et al. Early lactate clearance is associated with improved outcome in severe sepsis and septic shock. Crit Care Med 2004;32(8):1637–42.

52. Pan J, Peng M, Liao C, et al. Relative efficacy and safety of early lactate clearance-guided therapy resuscitation in patients with sepsis: a meta-analysis. Medicine (Baltimore) 2019;98(8):e14453.

53. Nguyen HB, Loomba M, Yang JJ, et al. Early lactate clearance is associated with biomarkers of inflammation, coagulation, apoptosis, organ dysfunction and mortality in severe sepsis and septic shock. J Inflamm (Lond) 2010;7:6.

54. Chertoff J, Chisum M, Simmons L, et al. Prognostic utility of plasma lactate measured between 24 and 48 h after initiation of early goal-directed therapy in the management of sepsis, severe sepsis, and septic shock. J Intensive Care 2016;4:13.

55. Jones AE, Shapiro NI, Trzeciak S, et al, Emergency Medicine Shock Research Network (EMShockNet) Investigators. Lactate clearance vs central venous oxygen saturation as goals of early sepsis therapy: a randomized clinical trial. JAMA 2010;303(8):739–46.

56. Tisherman SA, Barie P, Bokhari F, et al. Clinical practice guideline: endpoints of resuscitation. J Trauma 2004;57(4):898–912.

57. Davis JW, Kaups KL, Parks SN. Base deficit is superior to pH in evaluating clearance of acidosis after traumatic shock. J Trauma 1998;44:114–8.

58. Mutschler M, Nienaber U, Brockamp T, et al, TraumaRegister DGU. Renaissance of base deficit for the initial assessment of trauma patients: a base deficit-based classification for hypovolemic shock developed on data from 16,305 patients derived from the TraumaRegister DGU®. Crit Care 2013;17(2):R42.

59. Gale SC, Kocik JF, Creath R, et al. A comparison of initial lactate and initial base deficit as predictors of mortality after severe blunt trauma. J Surg Res 2016; 205(2):446–55.

60. Kulkarni AP, Kothekar AT, Divatia JV. Textbook of hemodynamic monitoring and therapy in the critically ill. New Delhi, India: Jaypee Brothers Medical Publishing; 2019.
61. Marino P. The ICU Book, 4th edition P. In: Section IV. Disorders of circulatory flow. Philadelphia, PA: Wolters Kluwer, Lippincott Williams & Wilkins; 2014. p. 193–279.
62. Darovic GO, Simonelli R. Pharmacologic influences on hemodynamic parameters. Hemodynamic monitoring: invasive and non-invasive clinical application. 3rd edition 2002. p. 305–45. Philadelphia, PA: Sanders.
63. Available at: https://accessdata.fda.gov/drugsatfda_docs/label/2017/209360s000lbl.pdf. Accessed February 21, 2021.
64. Available at: https://dosing.giapreza.com. Accessed February 21, 2021.

Resuscitation of the Traumatically Injured Patient

Kristen M. Burton-Williams, MSN, APRN, ACCNS-AG, CCRN-K, TCRN, FCNS

KEYWORDS

- Trauma resuscitation • Permissive hypotension • Damage control resuscitation
- Shock • Crystalloid • Blood

KEY POINTS

- Early identification of injuries and prompt treatment offer the best chances of survival.
- Primary and secondary assessments offer the most reliable means of identifying injuries. Injury patterns can be predicted based on known mechanisms.
- A lethal triad of metabolic acidosis, hypothermia, and trauma-induced coagulopathy must be anticipated and treated for the best possible outcome for the patient.
- Shock states causing inadequate tissue perfusion are a precursor to the lethal triad and require immediate intervention using the most current evidence-based practices including permissive hypotension.
- Special consideration must be given to the geriatric and obstetric population.
- Lessons learned from the military include the use of damage control resuscitation to achieve hemodynamic stability while controlling components of the lethal triad, delaying definitive surgical treatment, and using tranexamic acid to prevent and treat excessive blood loss.

INTRODUCTION

Trauma affects people of all ages. According to the most recent data available from the Centers for Disease Control branch of vital statistics, trauma is the fourth leading cause of death among all ages in the United States, and the leading cause of death in people aged 1 to 44 years.[1] A strong body of evidence demonstrates that treatment rendered in the early stages after injury has the greatest impact on the patient's outcome.

Advanced Trauma Life Support (ATLS) has provided the fundamental framework for rapid assessment and resuscitation of the injured patient since 1978. The overarching principle is based on the concept that a lethal reproducible pattern occurs among

593 Eddy Street, Providence, RI 02903, USA
E-mail address: Kristen.burton-williams@lifespan.org

Crit Care Nurs Clin N Am 33 (2021) 245–261
https://doi.org/10.1016/j.cnc.2021.05.002
0899-5885/21/© 2021 Elsevier Inc. All rights reserved.
ccnursing.theclinics.com

patients with severe trauma. Early identification and treatment offer the best chance of survival.[2] The ATLS algorithms provide standardized, evidence-based guidelines for the treatment of trauma patients.[3]

BLUNT VERSUS PENETRATING

Mechanisms of injury for trauma patients can be divided into blunt trauma and penetrating trauma. Blunt trauma is an injury to the body caused by forceful impact, injury, or physical collision with a dull object or surface. Blunt trauma most often occurs in motor vehicle collisions and falls. In motor vehicle collisions, rapid deceleration causes the body to push into the dashboard, steering wheel, or seatbelt. Common injuries resulting include contusions, abrasions, fractures, and damage to internal organs.[3]

Penetrating injury is the result of abrupt, direct application of a mechanical force in which an object or surface pierces the body, causing an open wound. Tissue damage is usually localized to the path of penetration. The severity of the injury is dependent on the organs and/or vessels penetrated.[3,4]

INITIAL MANAGEMENT

Initial management of the traumatically injured patient includes a rapid primary survey with simultaneous resuscitation, secondary survey, and definitive care. The primary survey identifies life-threatening conditions in a prioritized sequence based on the degree of threat. The abnormality posing the greatest threat to life is addressed first. The primary survey follows the ABCDE sequence of airway, breathing, circulation, disability, environment/exposure (**Table 1**).

The secondary survey includes a complete head to toe physical examination and evaluation of the patient's history. It is important to note the secondary survey does not begin until the primary survey is complete, resuscitative efforts are initiated, and vital functions are normalized. Trauma patients require frequent re-evaluation of the clinical condition always beginning with the primary survey to ensure new findings are not overlooked and to identify deterioration in previously noted findings.

During the secondary survey, a detailed history of the patient is obtained using the allergies, medications, past medical history, last time of PO intake, events leading to incident, tetanus status (AMPLET) pneumonic (**Table 2**). A patient's condition is greatly influenced by mechanism of injury, so knowing the circumstances of the injury or events leading up to the injury can narrow a patient's diagnosis. Some injuries can be presumed or predicted based on mechanism or whether an injury was caused by blunt or penetrating force.[3]

DEFINITIVE CARE

Definitive care describes the range of treatments that can be administered in a health care facility to provide the necessary level of trauma care to meet the patient's needs. Trauma Centers across the United States are verified by the American College of Surgeons to evaluate and improve trauma care. Trauma Center Levels range from I-V, providing comprehensive care from prevention through rehabilitation through initial evaluation and stabilization, respectively. Levels are determined by resource availability, capability, readiness, and performance improvement.[3,5]

Patient outcomes are directly related to the time elapsed between injury and properly delivered definitive care. Therefore, evaluation and decision to transfer to a higher level trauma center should occur within the first 15 to 30 minutes of arrival.[6] Patients experiencing signs of shock, significant physiologic deterioration, or progressive

Table 1
Primary survey C-ABCDE

Recognize	Assessment	Management
C Catastrophic bleeding	Assessing for life-threatening hemorrhage	• Apply direct pressure compression bandage • Tourniquet for extremity bleeding (note time applied)
A Airway maintenance with cervical spine immobilization	Airway patency, tracheal position, mental status to support airway protection	• Cervical immobilization avoiding excessive movement. Always suspect spinal injury exists until proven otherwise. • Frequent evaluation of airway, monitoring for progressive airway loss. If intubation is contraindicated, a surgical airway should be established.
B Breathing and ventilation	Expose patient's neck and chest. Visually inspect and palpate to assess jugular venous distention, chest wall expansion, crepitus, hematomas, or direct injuries to the chest wall	• All injured patients should receive supplemental oxygen with hemoglobin saturation monitoring. Injuries that significantly impair ventilation include tension pneumothorax, massive hemothorax, open pneumothorax, and tracheal or bronchial injuries. These injuries often require immediate attention to ensure effective ventilation. Because a tension pneumothorax compromises ventilation and circulation, chest decompression should be immediately performed when clinically suspected.
C Circulation with Hemorrhage Control	Assess Level of Consciousness (LOC): skin perfusion (color, temperature, mottling, capillary refill), quality of pulse. Physical assessment includes inspecting areas for potential large volume blood loss such as chest, abdomen, retroperitoneum, pelvis and long bones. A focused assessment with sonography for trauma (FAST exam) is recommended.	• Establish vascular access (IV, 10). Goal is to replace intravascular volume. • Identify and stop external bleeding with direct pressure, or tourniquet Be mindful of risk for ischemic injury with prolonged tourniquet use. • Immediate stabilization including chest decompression, pelvic stabilization and extremity splinting until definitive management is established.

(continued on next page)

Table 1
(continued)

Recognize	Assessment	Management
D Disability	Perform a rapid neurologic assessment Assess: AVPU • Alert • Verbal • Painful stimuli • Unresponsive Assess: Glascow Coma Scale (GCS) • Pupil size and reaction, motor response, verbal response	• Limit noise and stimulus during examination. Darken area to inspect pupils. • Be prepared to provide osmotic therapy, assist with insertion of an external ventricular drainage (EVD) system during secondary survey.
E Exposure or environmental control	Completely undress patient to perform a thorough examination and identify injuries while preventing hypothermia.	• Use commercially approved warming devices when administering IV fluid or blood. • Prewarm patient's room if possible. • Use warm blankets and minimize exposure.

Content derived from: American College of Surgeons Committee on Trauma. (2018). Advanced Trauma Life Support (ATLS) Student Course Manual. (10). Chicago. Illinois. United States of America.[3]

Table 2 Secondary survey	
A	Allergies
M	Medications currently used
P	Past illness, medical and surgical history, pregnancies
L	Last meal
E	Events/Environment surrounding trauma event
T	Tetanus status

Content derived from: American College of Surgeons Committee on Trauma. (2018). Advanced Trauma Life Support (ATLS) Student Course Manual. (10). Chicago, Illinois, United States of America.[3]

deterioration in neurologic status require the highest level of care, and their outcome will be optimized from timely transfer.[3]

When a patient's treatment needs exceed the capability of the receiving institution, transfer should be considered. This decision requires a detailed assessment of the patient's injuries and knowledge of the capabilities of the institution, including equipment, resources, and personnel. Interhospital transfer guidelines will help determine the appropriate setting based on patient condition. These guidelines consider the patient's physiologic status, obvious injury, mechanisms of injury, comorbidities, and other factors that can affect the patient's prognosis.

The need for intervention before patient transfer requires expert clinical judgment. There are few exceptions that may warrant a delay in transfer of a patient to definitive care, including life-threatening injuries. These should be treated before patient transport if resources are available, and the necessary procedures, including operative intervention, can be performed quickly to ensure that the patient is in the best possible condition for transfer.[3]

LETHAL/TRAUMA TRIAD

Severely injured patients sustaining significant blood loss often develop the lethal "triad" of metabolic acidosis, hypothermia, and coagulopathy, ultimately producing irreversible shock (**Fig. 1**).[7] The components of the triad are interrelated. The triad results from tissue injury, hypoperfusion, and decreased oxygen delivery causing acidosis. This contributes to coagulopathy, which is perpetuated by hemodilution (often from excessive fluid administration), hypothermia, and the body's inflammatory

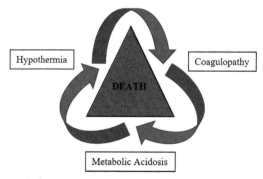

Fig. 1. Lethal/trauma triad.

response. Platelet (PLT) and coagulation factors are consumed, pH drops, and body temperature decreases.[8] Throughout the lethal triad, each condition contributes to a progressively worsening cycle that further aggravates coagulopathy (see **Fig. 1**).

METABOLIC ACIDOSIS

Metabolic acidosis is a result of shock-induced tissue hypoperfusion and hypoxia. It is a priority to treat the underlying condition to avoid this deadly complication. In the absence of oxygen, anabolic metabolism occurs. A byproduct of anabolic metabolism is lactic acid, which precipitates metabolic acidosis. Metabolic acidosis can also be induced by chloride infusion, which is described later in this article.

Acidosis has also been shown to inhibit the propagation phase of thrombin generation, accelerate fibrinogen degradation,[8] and adversely affect clotting factors II, V, VIIa, and X. It may be seen clinically as increasing prothrombin time (PT) and partial thromboplastin time values.[9] The clinical focus for the treatment of acidosis-induced coagulopathy must be on prevention because acidosis-induced coagulopathy cannot be acutely corrected by pH neutralization.[10]

Resuscitation is not complete until acidosis is resolved. Traumatically injured patients may experience occult hypoperfusion. In occult hypoperfusion, vital signs remain normal, but the patient will have a persistently elevated serum lactate level, evident of persistent anabolic metabolism. End points of resuscitation are achieved when tissue perfusion is restored.

HYPOTHERMIA

Clinical hypothermia defined as a core temperature ≤35° C is independently associated with increased mortality and may directly interfere with hemostatic processes by slowing down activity of coagulation enzymes and is associated with increased blood loss and the transfusion of more blood products.[10–12]

Hypothermia is exacerbated by exposure, fluid resuscitation, evaporation, sedatives, paralytics, alcohol, and illicit substances. Hypothermia results in vasoconstriction and decreased heart rate (HR) and cardiac output (CO), which further impairs tissue perfusion. Hypothermia also blunts the inflammatory response, causing decreased PLT function, increased fibrinolysis, and reduced clotting activity.

Hypothermia can be present on arrival or may develop throughout the admission, and strategies to prevent hypothermia should begin in the prehospital setting. Prevention measures include avoiding overexposure to elements and ambient temperatures, rapid extrication and transport, use of thermal blankets, and warmed fluid administration.[13]

Accidental hypothermia on the emergency department is frequently observed in trauma patients. The temperature of resuscitation area should be increased to minimize loss of body heat. In emergencies, patients are exposed for assessment, and fluids are often rapidly administered at room temperature, contributing to a drop in body temperature. The primary intervention to treat and prevent hypothermia is to control hemorrhage. Supplementary interventions include the use of warm blankets and infusion warmers for blood products and resuscitative fluids and maintaining a warm ambient room temperature.[3,10,11]

A multicenter retrospective cohort study was performed in adult trauma patients admitted to the intensive care unit (ICU) of two level-1 trauma centers between 2007 and 2012. Hypothermia was defined as a core body temperature of ≤35°C. Logistic regression analyses were performed to quantify the effect of hypothermia on 24-hour and 28-day mortality and to develop a prediction model.

Patients were divided into a normothermic or hypothermic group. Of a total of 953 patients admitted to the ICU, 354 (37%) patients had hypothermia. Hypothermia was associated with a significantly increased mortality at 24 hours and 28 days. The hypothermic group was more severely injured, coagulopathic, acidotic, and had higher mortality rates. Almost 50% of the patients who died within 28 days had a core body temperature lower than 32°C on admission to the ICU.[12]

Rewarming to a core temperature of 36°C to 37°C is advisable before transfer unless the patient is stable and achieved temperature homeostasis. This will ensure adequate warming before transferring the patient to another unit. However, rewarming should cease after 37°C because temperatures in this range are also associated with poor outcome and increased mortality.[14]

TRAUMA-INDUCED COAGULOPATHY

Trauma-induced coagulopathy (TIC) is present in 25% to 35% of trauma patients upon arrival to the hospital. The pathophysiology of TIC is multifaceted and is understood to primarily be caused by inflammatory and metabolic changes produced immediately after injury from both tissue hypoperfusion and direct tissue injury.[9]

Coagulopathy as a result of consumption of clotting factors and disseminated intravascular coagulation (DIC) is a primary mechanism of TIC. Patients in DIC experience a nonsurgical bleeding from muscle regions and wounds. DIC is characterized by systemic intravascular activation of coagulation, resulting in thrombin generation in the systemic circulation that can originate from and cause damage to the endothelium and microvasculature. Coagulopathy can also result from hemodilution of coagulation factors from blood lost and resuscitative fluids administered. Inactivation of clotting factors occurs secondary to hypothermia, which triggers the release of tissue factors with anticoagulant effects. Coagulopathy contributes to worsening hemorrhage and contributes to poor perfusion and acidosis. Treatment of coagulopathy is ultimately achieved when the bleeding has stopped. This can be aided by application of hemostatic dressings, replacement of PLTs and clotting factors, and screening for DIC.[8,10,11]

VISCOELASTIC ASSAYS

Standard coagulation tests are often inadequate to identify acute coagulopathy from shock because they identify early phases of clot formation only. Viscoelastic assays, thromboelastography (TEG), and rotational thromboelastometry (ROTEM) are emerging alternatives for point-of-care testing that may aid in early coagulopathy detection. Standard coagulation tests such as PT, activated partial thromboplastin, international normalized ratio, fibrinogen, and PLT count are performed. These tests only evaluate the initiation of the hemostatic process and are ineffective in evaluating the viscoelastic properties of whole blood. TEG/ROTEM allows for a more qualitative analysis of the individual cellular components and their interactions. Although there is evidence to support transfusion therapy guided by TEG/ROTEM reduces perioperative and postoperative bleeding and transfusion requirements, more clinical studies are needed in this area. Owing to the lack of high-quality evidence and unclear parameters for testing, clinicians should exercise caution in the application of these tests.[15,16]

SHOCK

Shock is a phenomenon of impaired perfusion at the cellular level and has been described historically as, "a momentary pause in the act of death."[17] Shock is characterized by clinical evidence of decreased perfusion and failure of adequate oxygen delivery to vital tissues and organs in relation to their metabolic needs. Failure to reverse shock will ultimately result in death. Time is the essence for the successful management of shock and begins with early recognition.[3,18,19]

The second step, which often occurs simultaneously with shock recognition, is to identify the cause of shock and treat accordingly. Categories of shock include hypovolemic, distributive, obstructive, cardiogenic, and neurogenic. Trauma patients may experience shock due to a variety of causes. For example, a patient may experience tension pneumothorax or cardiac tamponade leading to obstructive shock. Patients with a high-level spinal cord injury may experience neurogenic shock. It is critical that the clinician is able to differentiate between shock states and identify the cause so that appropriate treatments can be implemented.

Hypovolemic shock occurs when the circulatory volume is depleted from blood or fluid losses. Hypovolemic shock may be classified as hemorrhagic shock versus nonhemorrhagic. Nonhemorrhagic hypovolemic shock may be caused by digestive losses such as vomiting, diarrhea, or nasogastric suction. Renal losses may be attributed to conditions causing polyuria such as a traumatic head injury.

Distributive shock occurs because of inappropriate vasodilatation of the peripheral blood vessels from sepsis, anaphylaxis, drug reactions, endocrine, and neurogenic abnormalities. Patients require prompt identification and treatment of the underlying problem, and fluid resuscitation with vasopressor support.

Obstructive shock is associated with obstruction of the heart or the great vessels. Tension physiology, as in tension pneumothorax/hemothorax and cardiac tamponade, leads to high pressure in the chest, either in the hemithorax or pericardial sac, respectively. This effectively obstructs venous return and diminishes cardiac output leading to inadequate perfusion. Immediate intervention is required to decompress the pressure in the chest, allowing for uncongested blood flow.

Cardiogenic shock is failure of the "pump" and may arise from acute coronary syndrome (ACS), mechanical failure, and/or arrhythmias. Prompt evaluation of an electrocardiogram (EKG) and/or transesophageal echocardiogram (TEE) will help clinicians focus their treatment and determine if assistive devices such as an left ventricular assistive device (LVAD) or pacemaker are required. Intravenous fluids are used judiciously, and vasopressors may be initiated for concern for hypoperfusion.

Neurogenic shock is caused by injury to the spinal cord and may lead to a form of vasogenic shock. This is estimated to occur in up to 20% of cervical spine injuries. The damage to the spinal cord, in effect, leads to a sympathectomy, where the sympathetic nerve along the spine is disrupted, preventing nerve signals from passing through. This results in bradyarrhythmias, inappropriate vasodilation, and resultant hypotension and temperature dysregulation. This form of vasoplegic shock is to be differentiated from spinal shock—a temporary loss or reduction of motor and sensory function after injury to the spinal cord.[3,20,21]

One of the most common types of shock in trauma patients is hemorrhagic shock.

In hemorrhagic shock, loss of circulating volume leads to decreased preload and decreased stroke volume. This results in a compensatory release of catecholamines resulting in a progressive increase in HR and vasoconstriction. Owing to these compensatory mechanisms, a normal blood pressure (BP) is initially maintained; however, perfusion is altered because of the decreased circulating volume. As circulating volume continues to decline, HR continues to increase, and vasoconstriction continues. Eventually, compensatory mechanisms fail, resulting in hypotension and perfusion declines. Severity of hemorrhagic shock is divided into four classes, described in **Table 3**.

Volume repletion provides only temporary benefit until bleeding has stopped. In hemorrhagic shock, oxygen delivery depends on cardiac output rather than BP.[21,22] The most effective method of restoring adequate CO, end-organ perfusion, and tissue oxygenation is to restore venous return, which is ultimately achieved by locating and stopping the source of bleeding.[3,18]

Astute physical assessment is key in identifying early signs of hypoperfusion. Decreased perfusions states may manifest as cool extremities, diaphoresis, delayed capillary refill, and decreased urine output. Increasing HR, decreasing pulse pressure, and tachypnea are early signs while decreased BP is a late sign of hypoperfusion. Hemorrhage control and balanced fluid resuscitation should be initiated when early signs and symptoms of blood loss are apparent or suspected and not be delayed until the BP is falling or absent. Refer to **Table 3** to see comparative clinical presentations in relation to hypovolemic shock states.

The goals of treating hemorrhagic shock include definitive control of hemorrhage and restoration of circulating volume. Hemorrhage control can be achieved by application of pressure to the direct site, the use of compressive and hemostatic dressings, pelvic binders, tourniquet application, and surgical intervention. Resuscitative endovascular balloon occlusion of the aorta (REBOA) is another method of hemorrhage control gaining more widespread use in patients with traumatic noncompressible torso hemorrhage. In this procedure, the aorta is occluded in one of three zones to prevent exsanguination from injuries distal to the balloon.[23] A meta-analysis by Manzano and colleagues, 2017, noted a positive effect on mortality rates in patients who received REBOA compared with an emergent thoracotomy in patients with noncompressible torso hemorrhage.[23,24]

SPECIAL CONSIDERATIONS
Older Adults

Older adults (OAs) present unique challenges. The effect of changes in anatomy and physiology and the impact of pre-existing medical conditions will influence outcomes. Common mechanisms of injury for OAs include falls, motor vehicle collisions, burns, and penetrating injuries. The primary survey sequence and resuscitation are the same as for younger adults; however, the timing, magnitude, and end points will be influenced by the unique anatomy and physiology of older patients.[3]

OAs experience decreased physiologic reserve and often fail to elicit compensatory responses. Aging causes arterial stiffness and decreased left ventricular (LV) compliance. Hypovolemia decreases preload, causing ventricles to underfill with a disproportionate drop in cardiac output. OAs may not be able to mount a tachycardic response to hemorrhage because of beta blockade, medications, and pacer dependence.

Hypervolemia increases risk of pulmonary edema due to decreased LV compliance. Therefore, echocardiography is recommended to assess fluid requirements in this population. Clear fluid administration should be limited to 20 mL/kg, with early administration of blood products to achieve a goal Hgb greater than 9 g/dL and mean arterial pressure >70 mm Hg.[25] In younger adults, initial fluid resuscitation is limited to 1-2 L to achieve a goal systolic blood pressure (SBP) of 80 to 90 mm Hg before initiation of blood products.

Early discussions regarding goals of care and treatment decisions are a patient-centered approach to care. Early and open dialog encourage communication with the patient and family. Oftentimes, patients have already discussed their wishes regarding life-sustaining measures before an acute event occurs. Early consultation

Table 3
Hemorrhagic shock classification

Symptoms	Stage I	Stage II	Stage III	Stage IV
Blood loss (% blood volume)	15	15–30	30–40	>40
Blood loss (mL)	750	750–1500	1500–2000	>2000
Heart rate (beats/min)	<100	>100	>120	>140
Blood pressure (mm Hg)	Normal	Normal	Reduced	Reduced
Breathing rate (resps/min)	14–20	20–30	30–40	>35
Consciousness	Low restless	Moderate restless	High restless, disorientation	Disorientation, lethargy

Content derived from: American College of Surgeons Committee on Trauma. (2018). Advanced Trauma Life Support (ATLS) Student Course Manual. (10). Chicago, Illinois, United States of America.[3]

with palliative care services may be helpful in determining goals of care and effective symptom management.

Medications

Medications may cause blunted responses to hemodynamic changes or exacerbate trauma physiology. Anticoagulation therapy, antiplatelet therapy, and the use of direct thrombin inhibitors, for example, pose significant problems for the bleeding patient. Identifying the type of drug and then administering a reversal agent, if available, may optimize patient outcomes. Medications that affect hemodynamics including beta-blockers, calcium channel blockers, angiotensin converting enzyme (ACE) inhibitors, angiotensin II receptor blockers, vasodilators, and others may blunt the anticipated hemodynamic response, causing atypical presentation and potential misdiagnosis or delayed diagnosis.

Pregnancy

It is important to note the following physiologic hemodynamic changes of pregnancy and take these into account when assessing perfusion status: Cardiac output increases by 1 to 1.5 L, HR increases by 10 to 15 beats per minute, and BP can be decreased by 5 to 15 mm Hg. In general, the best initial treatment for the fetus is to provide optimal resuscitation of the mother. The increase in CO is often influenced by the physical position the mother is in. Hypotension may result when mother is supine. Known as vena cava syndrome, fetal compression of the vena cava can cause a decrease in CO by 30% due to decreased venous return from the lower extremities. This is often alleviated by repositioning the mother and fetus, relieving uterine pressure on the inferior vena cava. Hypertension may be indicative of preeclampsia, an obstetric emergency requiring immediate intervention and expert consultation.[3] Although patients in pregnancy are treated in the same ATLS approach as nonpregnant patients, detailed discussion of assessment and management is outside the scope of this article.

Fluid Resuscitation

Traditionally, the goal of crystalloid fluid resuscitation was the achievement of normal SBP. New evidence supports a more conservative approach to fluid resuscitation because vigorous fluid resuscitation has been shown to increases the rate of uncontrolled hemorrhage, contributes to negative sequalae, and worsens survival.

Current ATLS recommendations include limiting crystalloid resuscitation to 1 to 2 L before initiating blood products.[3] Volume infused should be based on the patient's response to fluid administration focusing on evidence of adequate end-organ perfusion and tissue oxygenation. Urinary output of approximately 0.5 mL/h and downtrending lactic acid suggest adequate volume replacement. Although BP is an important measure, it does not adequately indicate tissue oxygenation and is often a late sign of hypoperfusion.

A study by Dutton in 2006 found that, after 30 minutes of infusion, 75% of fluid moves into interstitial space, leaving only 25% in vasculature.[18] Aggressive fluid resuscitation may lead to negative sequelae including acute respiratory distress syndrome, pulmonary and cerebral edema, compartment syndrome, and increased inflammatory response. Administration of crystalloid fluid also increases coagulopathy related to the binding of crystalloids to plasma proteins.[26] A detailed discussion of these sequalae is beyond the scope of this article.

One important consideration associated with crystalloid fluid resuscitation is the potential contribution to hyperchloremic acidosis.[27] In 2015, Barker reviewed and analyzed 4 studies investigating infusions of plasmalyte, 0.9% saline, and lactated ringer solution in the acute care setting. Studies varied in methodology, but data reflected complications of acidosis, acute kidney injury, or electrolyte disturbances associated with 0.9% saline infusions. Saline solution 0.9% has a pH 5.5 and is composed of 154 mEq/L of sodium and 154 mEq/L of chloride. Large-volume resuscitation with 0.9% saline causes acidosis by diluting serum bicarbonate. Chloride and bicarbonate ions adjust up and down reciprocally. Hyperchloremia leads to nonanion gap metabolic acidosis, often causing acute kidney injury.[28] Hyperchloremia in trauma patients compounds metabolic acidosis from injury associated with shock. Chloride partially regulates renal vascular resistance. High chloride concentrations cause renal vasoconstriction and decreased glomerular filtration rate, leading to renal complications.

Lactated ringer solution is the preferred fluid for trauma resuscitation as it closely mimics intravascular plasma and contains lower concentrations of sodium and chloride. Saline 0.9%, however, is often chosen for hemorrhagic resuscitation over lactated ringer solutions, as it is compatible and can be infused concurrently with blood products. Lactated ringer solution contains calcium, which affects the anticoagulant properties of citrate used in blood products and causes the blood to coagulate.[27]

PERMISSIVE HYPOTENSION

Permissive hypotension aims to maintain tissue perfusion while targeting lower BPs to avoid the dilution of coagulation factors, development of hypothermia, and increase in hydrostatic pressure. Reduced hydrostatic pressure limits the disruption of unstable, newly formed clots and secondary blood loss until hemostasis is achieved.[29] In addition, permissive hypotension has been shown to lessen postoperative coagulopathy and nonsurgical bleeding.[2] It is a conservative, physiologically guided approach and avoids risk of overload and further bleeding, improving patient outcomes by keeping the BP low enough to avoid exsanguination but still allow for end-organ perfusion.[20,30]

ATLS recommends permissive hypotension including limiting crystalloids to 1 to 2 L before transfusion of blood products and targeting SBP of 80 to 90 mm Hg. This is often counterintuitive for clinicians based on the concept that BP often indicates organ perfusion.

It is important to note that permissive hypotension is contraindicated in known and suspected in patients with head or spinal cord injuries. In this population, it is essential to maintain an SBP greater than 90 mm Hg to ensure cerebral perfusion and oxygenation and avoid secondary injury, including cerebral tissue death.[31–33]

EVIDENCE SUPPORTING PERMISSIVE HYPOTENSION

Bickell and colleagues studied the effects of delayed fluid resuscitation until time of operative intervention in hypotensive patients with penetrating torso injuries and found that delay of aggressive fluid resuscitation until operative intervention improves patient outcomes.[31] The study included 598 adults who presented with a prehospital SBP less than 90 mm Hg. Two hundred eighty-nine adults received delayed resuscitation versus immediate standard fluid resuscitation before reaching the hospital. Of the 289 who received delayed resuscitation, 203 (70%) survived, had a shorter length of stay, and discharged from the hospital alive. Of the patients who received immediate fluid resuscitation, 193 of 309 patients (62%) survived ($P = .04$). Both groups estimated intraoperative blood loss was similar.[31]

A clinical trial by Schreiber in 2015 assessed feasibility and safety of controlled resuscitation (CR) versus standard resuscitation (SR) in hypotensive trauma patients. All patients included in the study experienced an out-of-hospital SBP of 90 mm Hg or lower. The trial randomized 192 patients to either the CR group (n = 97) or the SR group (n = 95). Patients in the CR group received a 250-mL fluid bolus if no radial pulse was palpable or if the SBP was lower than 70 mm Hg. Additional 250-mL fluid boluses were given to maintain a palpable radial pulse or SBP 70 mm Hg or higher. Patients in the SR group received a 2L initial fluid bolus and additional fluid as needed to maintain SBP 110 mm Hg or greater. The protocol was maintained until 2 hours after hospital arrival or until hemorrhage control was achieved. Patients in the CR group received a mean crystalloid volume of 1L. Patients in the SR group received a mean crystalloid volume of 2.0 L in the SR group. Intensive care-free days, ventilator-free days, rate of renal injury, and rate of renal failure did not differ between groups. At 24 hours after admission, 5 deaths occurred in the CR group (5%), and 14 deaths occurred in the SR group (15%). Among patients with blunt trauma, 24-hour mortality rate was 3% in the CR group and 18% in the SR group with an adjusted odds ratio of 0.17 (95% confidence interval [CI], 0.03–0.92). Schreiber's study suggests that CR is achievable in out-of-hospital settings and may offer early survival advantages in blunt trauma.[34]

HEMOSTATIC RESUSCITATION

Hemostatic resuscitation aims at controlling coagulopathy in the bleeding trauma patient. Current hemostatic resuscitation recommendations include identifying the severity and primary product lost and replacing with equivalent volumes of specific product.

DAMAGE CONTROL RESUSCITATION

Damage control resuscitation (DCR) focuses on achieving hemodynamic stability in an unstable trauma patient by recognizing early coagulopathy and addressing all elements of the trauma triad concurrently.[35] Much of the evidence and trends in trauma care originate in the military and wartime practices. DCR is a concept from the military that has become common practice for use in the most severely injured civilian patients, attempting to prevent versus treat coagulopathy.[36] DCR challenges the traditional ATLS sequence of airway, breathing, and circulation and is advocating instead for a circulation-first approach.[19,37] Damage control involves massive transfusion (MT) of blood products. MT is described as a patient receiving more than 10 units of red blood cells (RBCs) in 24 hours or receiving more than 4 units of blood products in 1 hour.

DCR and MT are described by Holcomb and colleagues in the prospective, observational, multicenter, major trauma transfusion (PROMMTT)[38] and pragmatic randomized optimal platelet and plasma ratios (PROPPR) studies.[39]

The Prospective, Observational, Multi-center, Major Trauma Transfusion Study[38] was a prospective multi-institutional cohort study across ten US level I trauma centers. The association between in-hospital mortality, timing, and amount of blood products administered was assessed to determine the benefit of early transfusion of plasma and/or PLTs and time varying ratios of plasma to RBC transfusion and PLT to RBC transfusion in the massively transfused trauma patient. The results of the study suggested improved survival in first 6 hours as the ratio of transfused RBCs to plasma approached 1:1. Decreased mortality was associated with higher plasma and PLT ratios early in resuscitation.

The PROPPR study[39] is to date the largest multicenter prospective randomized control trial comparing a fresh frozen plasma (FFP) to PLT to RBC ratio of 1:1:1 and 1:1:2, respectively, in addition to standard of care interventions related to survival and all-cause mortality. The study involved 680 severely bleeding trauma patients who were assigned at random to control or intervention group (IG). The control group included 342 patients who received FFP, PLTs, and RBCs at a respective ratio of 1:1:2. The IG included 338 patients who received FFP, PLTs, and RBCs at a respective ratio of 1:1:1. The IG more rapidly achieved hemostasis and lower rate of death by exsanguination in the first 24 hours. There was no difference in overall survival rate at 24 hours and 30 days.

This study did identify limitations as excluding patients with brain injuries and becoming unblinded once the coolers arrived with the blood products. There was an increased use of plasma and PLTs transfused in the 1:1:1 group; however, no other safety differences were identified between the 2 groups.[39]

WHOLE BLOOD

Historically, whole blood was the primary blood product used to treat hemorrhagic shock.

Although transfusion whole blood is no longer a mainstream treatment, there is a resurgence of its use in both military and civilian settings to treat life-threatening bleeding. Whole blood is less available in civilian settings and therefore rarely transfused in the setting of hemorrhagic shock. There are recent data to suggest that whole-blood transfusion is associated with improved or comparable survival rates compared with resuscitation with blood product components.[40,41]

TRANEXAMIC ACID

Tranexamic acid (TXA) is an antifibrinolytic agent that binds and inhibits plasmin to stop fibrin breakdown and an emerging therapy to potentially treat or prevent excessive blood loss. Although used inconsistently across the United States, TXA is a part of MT protocols in over 60% of trauma centers.[42]

TXA should be given as early as possible but within 3 hours after injury. Delay in administration after trauma reduces its efficacy and may cause patient harm. Patients who have received TXA should be evaluated with ultrasound technology for abnormal clotting after 30 days of administration.

The Clinical Randomization of an Antifibrinolytic in Significant Hemorrhage-2 (CRASH-2) trial assessed effects of early administration of TXA on death, vascular occlusive events, and blood transfusion in trauma patients with significant hemorrhage. The large, randomized control trial included 274 hospitals in 40 countries. In this double-blinded study, 20,211 adult trauma patients with or at risk of significant bleeding were randomized within 8 hours of injury to either receive TXA or placebo. Researchers analyzed 10,060 patients who received TXA versus 10,067 who received placebo. Deaths due to bleeding were 1063 (35%), with the effect varying according to the time from injury to treatment. Early treatment ($\leq$1 hour after injury) significantly reduced risk of death due to bleeding198/3747 (5.3%) in the TXA group versus 286/3704 (7.7%) in the placebo group. Treatment 3 hours after injury increased risk of death due to bleeding by 4.4% versus 3.1% without treatment.

TXA administration was found associated with a reduction in all-cause mortality (14.5% vs 16%, P <.001). Findings from this study demonstrate that TXA is to be administered as early as possible to bleeding trauma patients and may be less effective and could be harmful if administered late after injury.[43]

The Military Application of Tranexamic Acid in Trauma Emergency Resuscitation (MATTERs) study[44] sought to characterize the use of TXA in combat injury by assessing the effectiveness of administration on total blood product use, thromboembolic complications, and mortality. This retrospective observational study compares TXA administration with no TXA administration in patients who receive at least 1 unit of packed RBCs. A subset of patients receiving MT ($\geq$10 units of packed RBCs) was also analyzed.

Of 896 consecutive admissions with combat injury, 293 received TXA. The TXA group had lower unadjusted mortality than no TXA (17.4% vs 23.9%, respectively; P = .03). The greatest benefit was to those who received MT (14.4% vs 28.1%, respectively; P = .004). The use of TXA was independently associated with improved survival (odds ratio = 7.228; 95% CI, 3.016–17.322) and less coagulopathy (P = .003).[44]

SUMMARY

Trauma is a leading cause of death, and treating a trauma patient requires a coordinated effort to achieve the best possible outcomes. Providers must be prepared to act in an organized and methodical manner. Recognizing and immediately treating causes of shock after trauma is a priority. Evidence from military research has supported improvements in practices in the care of patients with hypovolemia and hemorrhagic shock.

Practitioners must be skilled at recognizing signs of shock. Trauma victims may lose a significant amount of blood without showing overt clinical signs of shock. Internal blood loss may not be visible and is a significant threat to the trauma patient. In addition, a significant volume of blood may be lost before the patient develops hypotension. Therefore, practitioners must be able to recognize earlier signs of shock so that appropriate interventions can be implemented.

Treatment priorities include stopping the bleeding, providing DCR, and monitoring and treating the patient for signs of shock. If the patient can be stabilized and avoid the lethal trauma triad, definitive surgical care can be achieved for the far more stable patient when appropriate.

CLINICS CARE POINTS

- Early identification of injuries and prompt treatment offer the best chances of survival.

- Advanced Trauma Life Support has guided the standardized algorithms used to treat trauma victims since 1978.
- Primary and secondary assessments offer the most reliable means of identifying injuries. Injury patterns can be predicted based on known mechanisms.
- A lethal triad of metabolic acidosis, hypothermia, and trauma-induced coagulopathy must be anticipated and treated for the best possible outcome for the patient.
- Shock states causing inadequate tissue perfusion are a precursor to the lethal triad and require immediate intervention using the most current evidence-based practices including permissive hypotension.
- Special consideration must be given to the older adult and obstetric population.
- Lessons learned from the military include the use of damage control resuscitation to achieve hemodynamic stability while controlling components of the lethal triad, delaying definitive surgical treatment, and using tranexamic acid to prevent and treat excessive blood loss.

DISCLOSURE

This author has no financial or conflicts of interest to disclose.

REFERENCES

1. CDC. Injury prevention and control. 2018 2018. Available at: https://www.cdc.gov/injury/wisqars/LeadingCauses.html. Accessed December 5, 2020.
2. Dauer E, Goldberg A. What's new in trauma resuscitation. Adv Surg 2019;53:221–33.
3. American College of Surgeons Committee on Trauma. Advanced trauma life support (ATLS) student course manual. 10th ed. Chicago: American College of Surgeons; 2018.
4. Kuhajda I, Zarogoulidis K, Kougiomtzi I, et al. Penetrating trauma. J Thorac Dis 2014;6:461–5.
5. American Trauma Society. Trauma center levels explained. 2021. Available at: Trauma Center Levels Explained - American Trauma Society. amtrauma.org. Accessed January 2, 2021.
6. Leibner E, Andreae M, Galvagno S, et al. Damage control resuscitation. Clin Exp Emerg Med 2020;7:5–13.
7. Harrington D, Connolly M, Biffl W, et al. Transfer times to definitive care facilities are too long: a consequence of an immature trauma system. Ann Surg 2005;6:961–6.
8. Hess J, Brohi K, Dutton R, et al. The coagulopathy of trauma: a review of mechanisms. J Trauma 2008;65(4):748–54.
9. Bogert J, Harvin J, Cotton B. Damage control resuscitation. J Intensive Care 2016;31:177–86.
10. Martini W. Coagulation complications following trauma. Mil Med Res 2016;3:1–7.
11. Lapointe L, Von Rueden K. Coagulopathies in trauma patients. AACN Clin Issues 2002;13:192–203.
12. Balvers V, Van der Horst M, Graumans M, et al. Hypothermia as a predictor for mortality in trauma patients at admittance to the intensive care unit. J Emerg Trauma Shock 2016;9:97–102.
13. Paal G, Strapazzon G, Maeder B, et al. Accidental hypothermia-an update. Scand J Truama Resusc Emerg Med 2016;24:1–20.

14. Wade S, Salinas J, Eastridge B, et al. Admission hypo-or hyperthermia and survival after trauma in civilian and military environments. Int J Emerg Med 2011; 4:1–6.
15. Caspers M, Maegele M, Fröhlich M. Current strategies for hemostatic control in acute trauma hemorrhage and trauma-induced coagulopathy. Expert Rev Hematol 2018;11:987–95.
16. Veigas P, Callum J, Rizoli S, et al. A systematic review on the rotational thrombelastometry (ROTEM) values for the diagnosis of coagulopathy, prediction and guidance of blood transfusion and prediction of mortality in trauma patients. Scand J Trauma Resusc Emerg Med 2016;24:114.
17. Warren J. Surgical pathology and therapeutics. Philadelphia: W.B. Saunders; 1895.
18. Dutton R. Fluid management for trauma; where are we now? BJA Educ 2006;6: 144–7.
19. Petrosoniak A, Hicks C. Resuscitation resequenced: a rational approach to patients with trauma in shock. Emerg Med Clin North Am 2018;36:41–60.
20. Marik P, Weinmann M. Optimizing fluid therapy in shock. Curr Opin Crit Care 2019;25:246–51.
21. Strehlow M. Early identification of shock in critically ill patients. Emerg Med Clin North Am 2010;28:57–66.
22. Wo C, Shoemaker W, Appel P, et al. Unreliability of blood pressure and heart rate to evaluate cardiac output in emergency resuscitation and critical illness. Crit Care Med 1993;21:218–23.
23. Manzano N, Naranjo M, Foianini E, et al. A meta-analysis of resuscitative endovascular balloon occlusion of the aorta (REBOA) or open aortic cross-clamping by resuscitative thoracotomy in non- compressible torso hemorrhage patients. World J Emerg Surg 2017;12:1–9.
24. Brenner M, Bulger E, Perina D, et al. Joint statement from the American College of Surgeons Committee on Trauma (ACS COT) and the American College of Emergency Physicians (ACEP) regarding the clinical use of Resuscitative Endovascular Balloon Occlusion of the Aorta (REBOA). Trauma Surg Care Open 2018;3:1–3.
25. Ramesh G, Uma J, Farhath S. Fluid resuscitation in trauma: what are the best strategies and fluids? Int J Emerg Med 2019;12:1–6.
26. Boldt J. Fluid choice for resuscitation of the trauma patient: a review of the physiological, pharmacological, and clinical evidence. Can J Anaesth 2004;51: 500–13.
27. Barker M. 0.9% Saline induced hyperchloremic acidosis. J Truama Nurs 2015; 22(2):111–6.
28. Young J, Utter G, Schermer C, et al. Saline versus plasmalyte A in initial resuscitation of trauma patients. Ann Surg 2014;259:255–62.
29. Albreiki M. Permissive hypotensive resuscitation in adult patients with traumatic haemorrhagic shock: a systematic review. Eur J Trauma Emerg Surg 2018;44: 191–202.
30. Gourgiotis S, Gemenetzis G, Kocher H, et al. Permissive hypotension in bleeding trauma patients: helpful or not and when? Crit Care Nurse 2013;33:18–24.
31. Bickell W, Wall M, Pepe P, et al. Immediate versus delayed fluid resuscitation for hypotensive patients with penetrating torso injuries. N Engl J Med 1994;331: 1105–9.
32. Harris T, Thomas G, Brohi K. Early fluid resuscitation in severe trauma. BMJ 2012; 345:1–6.

33. Thompson M, McIntyre L, Hutton B, et al. Comparison of crystalloid resuscitation fluids for treatment of acute brain injury: a clinical and pre-clinical systematic review and network meta-analysis protocol. Syst Rev 2018;125:1–7.

34. Schrieber M, Meier E, Tisherman S, et al. A controlled resuscitation strategy is feasible and safe in hypotensive trauma patients: results of a prospective randomized pilot trial. J Trauma Acute Care Surg 2015;78:687–97.

35. Holcomb J, Jenkins D, Rhee P, et al. Damage control resuscitation: directly addressing the early coagulopathy of trauma. J Trauma 2007;62:307–10.

36. Datta R, Chatuvedi R. Fluid therapy in trauma. Med J Armed Forces India 2010; 66:312–6.

37. Ferrada P, Callcut R, Skarupa D, et al. Circulation first-the time has come to question the sequencing in the ABCs of trauma; an American Association for the Surgery of Trauma multicenter study. World J Emerg Surg 2018;13:8.

38. Holcomb J, Fox E, Wade C, et al. The prospective, observational, multicenter, major trauma transfusion (PROMMTT) study: comparative effectiveness of a time-varying treatment with competing risks. JAMA Surg 2013;148:127–36.

39. Holcomb J, Tilley B, Baraniuk S, et al. Transfusion of plasma, platelets, and red blood cells in a 1:1:1 vs a 1:1:2 ratio and mortality in patients with severe trauma: the PROPPR randomized control trial. JAMA 2015;313:471–82.

40. Jones A, Frazier S. Consequences of transfusing blood components in patients with trauma: a conceptual model. Crit Care Nurse 2017;37:18–31.

41. Spinella P, Cap A. Whole blood: back to the future. Curr Opin Hematol 2016;23: 536–42.

42. Jawa R, Singer A, Mccormack J, et al. Tranexamic acid use in United States trauma centers: a national survey. Am Surg 2016;82:439–47.

43. CRASH-2 trial collaborators, Roberts I, Shakur H, Afolabi A, et al. The importance of early treatment with tranexamic acid in bleeding trauma patients: an exploratory analysis of the CRASH-2 randomised controlled trial. Lancet 2011;377: 1096–101.

44. Morrison J, Dubose J, Rasmussen T, et al. Military Application of Tranexamic Acid in Trauma Emergency Resuscitation (MATTERs) study. Arch Surg 2012;147: 113–9.

Nursing Care for the Initial Resuscitation of Severe Sepsis Patients

Mary G. Carey, PhD, RN[a],*,
Emily Katherine Valcin, DNP, RN, CNL, CCRN-K[b],
David Lent, DNP, MS, RN, CNL, CCRN-K, PCCN-K[c],
Mackenzie White, MS, RN[d]

KEYWORDS

- Sepsis resuscitation • Nursing care • Hospitalization • Critical care

KEY POINTS

- Nurses play an important role in the early identification of potential sepsis for hospitalized patients.
- Although bacterial infections are the most common causes, fungal, viral, and protozoan infections also can lead to sepsis.
- Strategies for implementing Surviving Sepsis Campaign guidelines into nursing care include champions committed to reducing the incidence of sepsis, a culture of performance improvement for sepsis, and implementing guidelines as part of daily practice.

INTRODUCTION

In the United States, sepsis affects approximately 3 in 1000 people, and severe sepsis contributes to more than 200,000 deaths per year.[1] Among hospitalized people, sepsis is the most common cause of death.[2] Although it occurs in only approximately 2% of all hospitalizations, sepsis accounts for as many as 25% of intensive care unit (ICU) bed utilizations. Early identification of sepsis by nurses is critical because it is estimated that there is an 8% increase in the mortality rate for every hour of antibiotic treatment delay past onset of hypotension.[3–5] Thus, expert nursing knowledge and skills are required to identify the initial signs of deterioration from newly developed sepsis as well as the ongoing implementation of best evidence-based practice for the known sepsis patient.

[a] Clinical Nursing Research Center, University of Rochester Medical Center, 601 Elmwood Avenue, Rochester, NY 14642, USA; [b] University of Rochester Medical Center, 601 Elmwood Avenue, Rochester, NY 14642, USA; [c] Adult Critical Care Outcomes, University of Rochester Medical Center, 601 Elmwood Avenue, Rochester, NY 14642, USA; [d] Adult Critical Care, University of Rochester Medical Center, 601 Elmwood Avenue, Rochester, NY 14642, USA
* Corresponding author.
E-mail address: mary_carey@urmc.rochester.edu

Crit Care Nurs Clin N Am 33 (2021) 263–274
https://doi.org/10.1016/j.cnc.2021.05.003

DEFINING SEPSIS

Sepsis is described most simply as life-threatening organ dysfunction due to infection. Due to its complex, syndromic presentation, however, and the absence of a conclusive diagnostic test, defining sepsis has been an iterative and evolving process. From the first attempt, Sepsis-1, released in the early 1990s, to Sepsis-2 and the Surviving Sepsis Campaign (SSC), launched in 2002, the definition of sepsis largely was guided by the presence of multiple nonspecific symptoms described as systemic inflammatory response syndrome (SIRS). The most recent definition, Sepsis-3, published in 2016, emphasizes the sequential organ failure assessment (SOFA) to characterize the organ dysfunction and the SOFA to screen patients for sepsis. In the development of Sepsis-3, the pathophysiologic burden on the host is emphasized rather than the triggering pathogen, which helps to distinguish sepsis from an uncomplicated serious infection. In the following sections, the definition of sepsis and the evolution of treatment are explored to provide historical context for the developing nurse.

Sequential Organ Failure Assessment Score

The SOFA score is calculated by scoring a variety of physiologic parameters on a 0 to 3 scale to evaluate respiratory status, coagulation, liver function, cardiovascular function, central nervous system, and renal function. Risk of sepsis is denoted through an upward change in the total SOFA score of 2 or more points. The SOFA score is considered reliable and highly predictive of the presence of sepsis. Concerns about the SOFA score include difficulty in calculating related most often to a lack of critical patient data and the overall time needed to calculate the SOFA score. In response, the quick SOFA (qSOFA) was developed to both simplify the screening process when fewer data were available and to reduce the time needed to evaluate the potential for sepsis. The qSOFA utilizes just 3 data points: respiratory rate greater than or equal to 22 breaths per minute, change in mental status, and systolic blood pressure less than or equal to 100 mm Hg. When an element is present, 1 point is given, an aggregate score greater than or equal to 2 points indicates organ dysfunction and the potential for sepsis. Overall, the qSOFA is less sensitive than SOFA, but is easier to administer and has been validated as predictive measure of organ dysfunction.[6]

Since 1990, many terms have been utilized to describe severity of sepsis, including sepsis, severe sepsis, and septic shock. These definitions have changed over time and some no longer are considered useful because of difficulty in recognizing or lack of utility in driving treatments.[7] The treatment of sepsis also has changed over time as new evidence has been published. In the early 1990s, Sepsis-1 defined sepsis using nonspecific variables that collectively described SIRS. In the setting of known or suspected infection, SIRS focused primarily on the host's systemic inflammatory response and the presence of 1 or more physiologic variables. The severity of the host's inflammatory response then was delineated by the presence of 1 or more of SIRS criteria: sepsis, the presence of SIRS plus organ failure; severe sepsis; and septic shock, sepsis-induced hypotension despite adequate fluid resuscitation.[8] In 2001, a consensus panel elected to expand the diagnostic criteria, however, the 3 classifications of sepsis, severe sepsis, and septic shock remained largely unchanged.[9]

At that time, the best available evidence for treatment of severe sepsis and septic shock involved initiation of goal-directed therapy (GDT). This therapy was focused primarily on maintaining cardiac preload, afterload, and contractility to balance oxygen delivery with oxygen demand in septic patients.[10] Specific bundles of interventions to be completed within 3-hours and within 6-hours from the onset of sepsis were defined in Sepsis-2. Recently published studies have called into question the necessity of the 3-hour and 6-hour intervention bundles and have led to a shift to a 1-hour bundle focusing on the following elements:

1. Measuring serum lactate
2. Obtaining blood cultures
3. Administering antibiotics
4. Administering intravenous fluids (IVFs) 30 mL/kg for hypotension or elevated serum lactate
5. Administering vasopressors for hypotension that continues after administration of IVFs

As described previously, Sepsis-1 defined sepsis using nonspecific variables that collectively described SIRS. In the setting of known or suspected infection, SIRS focused primarily on the host's systemic inflammatory response and the presence of 1 or more physiologic variables: temperature greater than 38°C or less than 36°C, heart rate greater than 90/min, respiratory rate greater than 20/min or $Paco_2$ less than 32 mm Hg (4.3 kPa), and white blood cell count greater than 12,000/mm^3 or less than 4000/mm^3 or greater than 10% immature bands.[8] The severity of the host's inflammatory response then was delineated by the presence of 1 or more of SIRS criteria: sepsis; severe sepsis, the presence of SIRS plus organ failure; and septic shock, sepsis-induced hypotension despite adequate fluid resuscitation.[8] In 2001, a consensus panel elected to expand the diagnostic criteria; however, the 3 classifications of sepsis, severe sepsis, and septic shock remained largely unchanged.[9]

Early Identification of Sepsis

Understanding of sepsis pathology continues to evolve and, in 2016, the Society of Critical Care Medicine (SCCM) and the European Society of Intensive Care Medicine (ESICM) further redefined the consensus definition of sepsis (Sepsis-3) as a dysregulated host response to infection that leads to life-threatening organ dysfunction.[11] The new definition is an umbrella syndrome that includes numerous pathogens. Sepsis-3 eliminated the highly sensitive yet nonspecific SIRS criteria in favor of a more sepsis-specific SOFA and a shortened version, the qSOFA score. In the development of Sepsis-3, the pathophysiologic burden on the host is emphasized rather than the triggering pathogen, which helps distinguish sepsis from an uncomplicated serious infection. In doing so, not only do SOFA and qSOFA aid in the early detection of sepsis but also they help guide treatment, something SIRS did not.[11]

RISKS AND TREATMENT

Sepsis and septic shock continue to be major health care problems. Although mortality related to septic shock has been reduced slightly in the past decade, it remains high, at greater than 20%.[12] In 2008, as part of a global response to optimize care for this group of patients, evidence-based clinical practice guidelines were developed by the SSC, a joint collaboration between SCCM and ESICM. The guidelines, first published in 2008 and then revised in 2012, represented a shift away from the aforementioned GDT, toward protocolized resuscitation, focused on early administration of antibiotics, hemodynamic support, and appropriate fluid resuscitation. Bacterial infection is the most common cause of sepsis, but fungal, protozoan, and viral infections, including severe acute respiratory syndrome coronavirus 2, the virus that causes coronavirus disease, also can lead to sepsis.[6,13,14] Common locations for the primary infection include the lungs, brain, urinary tract, skin, and abdominal organs.[15] Risk factors include being very young or old, a weakened immune system from conditions such as cancer or diabetes, major trauma, and burn injuries.[16]

A comprehensive review of the medical management of patients with sepsis and septic shock was provided through SSC guidelines but the guidelines lack the specifics of nursing-focused care that are essential for optimal outcomes for these patients.[17] Foremost, the early identification and initiation of treatment are critical in improving patient outcomes with each hour of delay being associated with an increase in absolute mortality.[18] High-quality nursing is fundamental for the early identification and early implementation of care bundles for the known or suspected sepsis patients. Thus, an international group of interested experts was identified by the World Federation of Critical Care Nurses, a top organization for critical care nurses to provide guidance for nursing care of severe sepsis patients.

Recommendations: Nursing Care of Severe Sepsis Patients

The convergence of objectives scoring tools, such as the SOFA and qSOFA, and subjective nursing concern or worry highlights the essential role that bedside nurses play in the early identification and initiation of best evidence-based interventions for patients with sepsis. There are additional nursing considerations that complement the current guidelines. Among nursing care tasks, the World Federation of Critical Care Nurses made 63 nursing-specific recommendations in the categories of prevention, infection management, initial resuscitation including hemodynamic support, and supportive nursing care.[19] Sepsis prevention recommendations include enhanced education, accountability, surveillance of nosocomial infections, hand hygiene, and prevention of respiratory, central line–related, surgical site, and urinary tract infections. Infection management recommendations included infection source and transmission-based precautions. Recommendations related to initial sepsis resuscitation included improved recognition of the deteriorating patient, seeking further assistance, diagnosis of severe sepsis, and initiating early resuscitation measures. Important elements of hemodynamic support related to improved tissue oxygenation and macrocirculation; the circulation of blood to and from the organs, as distinguished from microcirculation; and the circulation of the blood in the smallest blood vessels.[20] Recommendations related to supportive nursing care included: nutrition, scrupulous oral and eye care, and pressure ulcer prevention and management. Specifically, the scope of this current review is related to the nursing care for the initial resuscitation of septic patients.

Nursing Care for the Initial Resuscitation of Sepsis

Is the nurse worried?

In a recently published study, nurses' pattern recognition and sense of worry provided important information for the detection of acute physiologic deterioration. Nurses were asked to record perception of patient potential for deterioration using a 5-point worry factor scale at the start of the shift and with any changes in condition. Of 492 potential deterioration events identified, 380 (77%) were confirmed by reviewers as true deterioration events. Accuracy rates were significantly higher in nurses with more than a year of experience (68% vs 79%, respectively; $P = .04$). The authors recommended inclusion of "nurse worried" language in the electronic medical record.[21] Accordingly, bedside nurses must trust their intuition that there is a change in the patient and also remain diligent in recognizing subtle but important physiologic signs and symptoms of sepsis (**Table 1**).

Table 1
Physiologic signs and symptoms of sepsis

1	Patches of discolored skin
2	Decreased urine output
3	Change in mental ability
4	Low platelet count
5	Difficulty breathing
6	Abnormal heart functions
7	Chills, secondary to decreased body temperature
8	Unconsciousness

Data from L GR. Early Recognition and Management of Sepsis in Adults: The First Six Hours. *Am Fam Physician.* 2013;1:44-53.

Recognizing deterioration and severe sepsis

Early recognition and diagnosis of sepsis are paramount to ensuring survival and good patient outcomes. With the advent of electronic medical records, health scientists are developing artificial intelligence algorithms that function as early warning systems, to alert nurses to worrisome clinical patterns. These algorithms have demonstrated higher accuracy than traditional human-calculated risk scores and have an advantage in that results are available in real time.[22] Early warning systems are most helpful in situations where subtle changes in 1 or more vital signs, such as increasing heart and respiratory rate accompanied by low-grade fever occur over time or across shifts (**Tables 2** and **3**). Independently, these changes easily may be overlooked; however, the early warning algorithm may recognize the change and alert the nurse, who then may assess for sepsis earlier than they may have otherwise. Despite this, a disadvantage of these methods is reliance on data that are input into the electronic health record and may be sensitive to variations in practice, such as the frequency of vital signs documentation.

Seeking assistance early

Effective management of sepsis is extremely demanding and requires a sense of urgency, in other words, an all-hands-on-deck mentality. Nurses often are the first members of an interdisciplinary team to identify sepsis and play an important role in mobilizing the team. Research has shown optimal patient outcomes occur when nurses implement evidence-based communication strategies to convey accurate and timely communication among the health care disciplines, for example, Situation, Background, Assessment, and Recommendation.[19] Nurses who that identify potential sepsis should communicate to providers the urgent need for assessment and, if deemed necessary, the implementation of prescriptive sepsis bundles that require intensive nursing care, for example, blood cultures, antibiotics, initial laboratory work, and possible need for vasopressor or fluid support. The urgency of these interventions as well as monitoring for potential complications, such as acute respiratory distress syndrome or multiple organ dysfunction syndrome, may require almost constant nursing interventions. Given these demands, it is imperative, should a patient's condition warrant, that the nurse-to-patient ratio is adjusted to allow nurses to complete resuscitation modalities and rescue patients from life-threatening sepsis. Depending on patient response, transfer to a higher level of care, such as an ICU, should be considered.

Table 2
Clinical manifestation of sepsis

System	Manifestation	Significance
Cardiac	Clammy, cold skin; hypotension poor capillary refill; tachycardia	• Shock results from redistribution of intravascular circulation and myocardial depression. • Hypotension as the initial presentation has 2-fold increase risk of death.
Constitutional	Diaphoresis; fevers or rigors; malaise; myalgia	• Fever is the most common manifestation.
Dermatologic	Abscess; cellulitis; ecchymosis or petechiae; necrotizing fasciitis Regional lymphadenopathy	• Distinguish from direct bacterial invasion, lesions secondary to sepsis (disseminated intravascular coagulation), lesions from vasculitis, or microemboli (endocarditis).
Endocrine	Hyperglycemia; hypoglycemia	• In patients with diabetes mellitus, hyperglycemia may be the first clue of an infection.
Gastrointestinal	Abdominal pain, decreased bowel sounds, diarrhea (bloody or nonbloody), distention, rigidity, upper gastrointestinal tract blood loss, vomiting	• Consider early imaging to rule out renal obstruction and later imaging for renal abscess. • Placental abruption and septic abortion should be considered in pregnant patients.
Hematologic	Anemia, leukocytosis or leukopenia, thrombocytopenia	• Neutropenia is uncommon but may occur in older patients and in those with chronic alcohol abuse. • Microangiopathic hemolytic anemia is a feature of disseminated intravascular coagulation. • Thrombocytopenia often precedes the development of disseminated intravascular coagulation.
Hepatic	Coagulopathy, abnormal results on liver function testing, jaundice	• Abnormalities may occur in disseminated intravascular coagulation. • Coagulation abnormalities may increase bleeding risk.
Neurologic	Headache, altered mental status ranging from mild disorientation and lethargy to coma	• Older patients may present with subtle agitation or irritation.

(continued on next page)

System	Manifestation	Significance
Table 2 *(continued)*		
Pulmonary	Upper: dysphagia, lymphadenopathy, sore throat, trismus Lower: consolidated auscultatory findings, cough, hypoxia, pleuritic chest pain, shortness of breath, tachypnea, or hyperventilation	• Acute lung injury and acute respiratory distress syndrome are late complications; mechanical ventilation may increase risk of bleeding.
Renal	Anuria, oliguria, urinary sediments (suggestive of acute tubular necrosis)	• Primary infection may be genitourinary, but hypoperfusion may lead to organ dysfunction (acute renal failure).

Adapted or reprinted with permission from Diagnostic Approach to Palpitations, February 15, 2005, Vol 71, No 4, American Family Physician Copyright © 2005 American Academy of Family Physicians. All Rights Reserved.

Initiating Early Resuscitation Measures

To optimize outcomes of patients in the initial phases of sepsis, skilled critical care nurses should implement best evidence-based practice promptly and obtain blood specimens to culture for pathogens and monitor lactate levels, administer the primary dose(s) of antibiotics or IVFs, utilize advanced oxygen therapies, and initiate of vasopressors in accordance with medical orders without delay. The literature supports initial resuscitation of patients with sepsis should be provided through the use of hospital-based rapid response systems, because early response has demonstrated efficacy in improving mortality outcomes in severe sepsis.[19,23] Once identified, septic patients should be transferred promptly to a higher level of care to ensure compliance with best evidence-based practice given the labor-intensive nature of the therapies for sepsis. Higher nurse-to-patient ratios with critically ill patients result in improved compliance with sepsis bundle elements and fewer complications among septic patients.[24] Only 2 actions in the bundle are ordinal, that is, blood cultures should be obtained before administration of antibiotics; the other actions are concurrent.

The Sepsis Six nursing bundle, adapted, SSC[19]

1. Administer high-flow oxygen.
2. Obtain blood cultures.
3. Administer intravenous antibiotics.
4. Start IVF resuscitation.
5. Monitor hemoglobin and lactate levels.
6. Monitor hourly urine output.

Table 3	
Strategies for implementing Surviving Sepsis Campaign guidelines into nursing practice[14]	
1	Identify nursing champions in leading initiative.
2	Integrate SSC as performance improvement initiative for critical care and medical-surgical unit.
3	Include guidelines during daily practice, for example, daily rounds

CASE STUDY
Proteus mirabilis Infection

A 66-year-old man presented to the emergency department with hematuria and clots in his long-term Foley catheter. The patient had a medical history significant for hemorrhagic stroke that limited his independence due to right-sided hemiparesis, a deep vein thrombosis with an inferior vena cava filter, and previous coronary artery bypass graft surgery. In regard to the current events of the COVID-19 pandemic, just because a patient is COVID positive or waiting for testing results does not mean sepsis can be ruled out.[25] In other words, COVID can co-occur with bacterial sepsis. During the initial assessment, the nurse identified that the patient had a slight cough, low-grade fever, and increased respiratory effort with an SpO_2 of 88%. The patient immediately was isolated for suspicion for COVID-19. After appropriately donning personal protective equipment (PPE), oxygen was administered at 2-L nasal cannula and a nasal swab obtained and tested for the infection COVID-19. Next, the Foley catheter was replaced, and urine and blood cultures were obtained with a high suspicion for bacteremia related to urinary infection. While waiting for the COVID-19 test results, early sepsis was identified and managed with the early GDT Sepsis Six nursing bundle. The patient was appropriately admitted to an ICU under COVID isolation and early GDT was accomplished within the prescribed timeframe. Later that day, the COVID test result was negative and precautions were removed. Over the subsequent week, the patient progressively improved from early sepsis caused by a urinary Proteus mirabilis infection secondary to his long-term catheterization. The most common clinical symptom of P mirabilis bacterial is urinary tract infections.

Vital Signs	Arterial Blood Gases	Laboratory Tests	Therapies and Monitoring
Day 1			
Maximum temperature 37.8C°, RR 24, heart rate 100, blood pressure 95/55, SpO_2 88% on room air	7.28	Blood cultures: Klebsiella pneumoniae both sets; urinalysis: P mirabilis and Klebsiella pneumonia	High-flow oxygen, intake and output, hemoglobin and hematocrit, fluid bolus, vancomycin, Zosyn, and Unasyn, straight tip catheter changed to coudé tip with urine meter bag
Day 2			
Maximum temperature 37.9C°, RR 22; heart rate 105, blood pressure 85/49, SpO_2 93%	7.32	White blood cell count, 39.6, and bands, 12%; lactate 6.2 (9.6); urinalysis: Enterococcus faecalis and P mirabilis and Providencia stuartii and Klebsiella pneumonia	Oxygen 2-L nasal cannula, intake and output, hemoglobin and hematocrit, norepinephrine, daptomycin, Zosyn and Unasyn; operating room cystoscopy, bilateral ureteral stent insertion

(continued on next page)

(continued)			
Vital Signs	Arterial Blood Gases	Laboratory Tests	Therapies and Monitoring
Days 3 to 5			
Within normal limits	Not indicated	Not indicated	Intake and output, hemoglobin and hematocrit, Zosyn, ceftriaxone
Days 6 to 7			
Within normal limits	Not indicated	Positive *Clostridium difficile*	Intake and output, hemoglobin and hematocrit, Vancomyocin

Case Study Clinical Questions

1. Is this patient in septic shock?

   Sepsis is a clinical continuum ranging from bacteremia through septicemia to septic shock. On day 1, identify the term that best describes the patient's condition and include the best qSOFA score to match his condition. The patient was displaying signs of septicemia because his blood pressure still was within a normal range and he had a low-grade fever. Inflammatory mediators and other signaling molecules, for example, histamine, were being released by the immune defense cells causing inflammation, resulting in the observed physiologic changes. His qSOFA score is 2, which is considered positive for organ dysfunction.

2. What impact did the COVID-19 pandemic have on this patient's care?

   The COVID-19 pandemic had an impact on the care of this patient in several ways, because symptoms of COVID-19 and sepsis are similar; both must be considered likely causes of the patient's symptoms until 1 or both are ruled out. Because COVID-19 is highly contagious, the patient spent the first part of his hospitalization in isolation, limiting the nurse's ability to assess the patient frequently and readily without donning and doffing PPE.

3. Which elements of best evidence-based practice did this patient receive?

   All the Sepsis Six nursing bundle elements were accomplished, including oxygen therapy, obtaining blood cultures, administration of intravenous antibiotics, IVF resuscitation, monitor hemoglobin and lactate, and hourly urine output.

Case Study Discussion

Overall, with the application of early GDT by skilled critical care nurses, the patient's septic condition responded to the treatment, which prevented further physiologic decline. Once the urine culture results were received, the patient's antibiotic coverage was narrowed, a driving principle of antibiotic stewardship, to prevent the development of antibiotic resistance.[26]

DISCUSSION

Sepsis is a serious acute condition, which, if it is identified early and managed aggressively, can have reduced morbidity or mortality. For best outcomes, septic patients need prompt normalization of macrohemodynamic parameters, for example, heart rate, blood pressure, and so forth. Nurses' role is early identification of sepsis and is key given their omnipresence in the care of hospitalized patients. Strategies for implementing SSC guidelines into nursing care include identifying champions committed to reduce the incidence of sepsis; creating a culture of performance improvement for sepsis, for example, hospital sepsis committees; and implementing guidelines as part of daily practice, for example, hospital rounds.[19]

Nursing Impact

Among health care workers, nurses spend the most time at the bedside and play a key role in advocating for optimal patient care. In the presence of a deteriorating patient, SSC guidelines should be considered because they have evidence to improve patient outcomes and survival.[27] The true crux of evidenced-based practice, however, is that nursing care should be tailored to meet the individual needs of a patient and not implemented in the absence of sound clinical judgment and consideration for the patient's preferences. In these situations, it is imperative that nurses understand the most up-to-date recommendations so they may best be applied for the benefit of patients.

Global Considerations

Lack of widespread knowledge in the effective management of sepsis makes it the number 1 preventable cause of death worldwide.[12] Sepsis mortality is as high as 50%; this high global mortality may be due to low vaccination compliance, suboptimal quality of hospital care, and lack of early sepsis recognition and treatment. Particularly in the wake of the COVID-19 pandemic, global considerations are warranted in regard to sepsis mortality. In 2012, the Global Sepsis Alliance, a nonprofit charity organization, launched the World Sepsis Day initiative that occurs annually on September 13, in an effort to raise awareness, improve sepsis care, and promote action across the globe. Remarkably, this initiative resulted in a 2017 recommendation by the World Health Assembly, the decision-making body of the World Health Organization, to provide formal recommendations and action steps, to assist nations in reducing the worldwide burden of sepsis for both children and adults.[28]

SUMMARY

Overall, sepsis mortality remains a serious global health problem; yet, early recognition of sepsis by nurses can reduce mortality, morbidity, and long-term consequences for patients. Educating nurses as to what steps to take when they recognize signs and symptoms in potentially septic patients can improve early treatment, especially when augmented by computer early warning systems that alert nurses of worrisome clinical patterns. Nurses should be familiar with the most up-to-date evidence-based protocols and anticipate the next step in care to minimize treatment delays. Finally, the nurse-to-patient ratio should be adjusted or patients should be transferred to a higher level of care, when possible, to better manage the increased demands of sepsis care.

CLINICS CARE POINTS

- Although bacterial infections are the most common causes of sepsis, fungal, viral, and protozoan infections also can lead to sepsis.
- Nurses' role is the early identification of sepsis is key given their omnipresence in the care of hospitalized patients.

- Strategies for implementing SSC guidelines into nursing care include champions committed to reducing the incidence of sepsis, a culture of performance improvement for sepsis, and implementing guidelines as part of daily practice.

DISCLOSURE

The authors have nothing to disclose.

REFERENCES

1. Seymour CW, Angus DC. Sepsis and septic shock. In: Jameson J, Fauci AS, Kasper DL, et al, editors. Harrison's Principles of Internal Medicine, 20e. McGraw Hill. Available at: https://nam03.safelinks.protection.outlook.com/?url=https%3A%2F%2Faccessmedicine.mhmedical.com%2Fcontent.aspx%3Fbookid%3D2129%26sectionid%3D192032122&data=04%7C01%7Cm.packiam%40elsevier.com%7Ca956bff3a77840bc4b1008d929c0d475%7C9274ee3f94254109a27f9fb15c10675d%7C0%7C0%7C637586731078112426%7CUnknown%7CTWFpbGZsb3d8eyJWIjoiMC4wLjAwMDAiLCJQIjoiV2luMzIiLCJBTiI6Ik1haWwiLCJXVCI6Mn0%3D%7C1000&sdata=X2hNsi2SuP9S3ufcx2vvuhJE49NjRFJOIsXeIS7bkuo%3D&reserved=0.
2. Deutschman CS, Tracey K. Sepsis: current dogma and new perspectives. Immunity 2014;40:463–75.
3. Kumar A, Roberts D, Wood KE, et al. Duration of hypotension before initiation of effective antimicrobial therapy is the critical determinant of survival in human septic shock. Crit Care Med 2006;34:1589–96.
4. Pruinelli L, Westra BL, Yadav P, et al. Delay within the 3-hour surviving sepsis campaign guideline on mortality for patients with severe sepsis and septic shock. Crit Care Med 2018;46:500–5.
5. Husabø G, Nilsen RM, Flaatten H, et al. Early diagnosis of sepsis in emergency departments, time to treatment, and association with mortality: an observational study. PLoS One 2020;15:e0227652.
6. Marik PE and Taeb AMJJoTD. SIRS, qSOFA and new sepsis definition. 2017. 2017;9:943-945.
7. Gül F, Arslantaş MK, Cinel İ, et al. Changing definitions of sepsis. Turk J Anaesthesiol Reanim 2017;45:129–38.
8. Bone RC, Balk RA, Cerra FB, et al. Definitions for sepsis and organ failure and guidelines for the use of innovative therapies in sepsis. The ACCP/SCCM consensus Conference committee. American College of chest Physicians/Society of critical care medicine. Chest 1992;101:1644–55.
9. Levy MM, Fink MP, Marshall JC, et al. 2001 SCCM/ESICM/ACCP/ATS/SIS international sepsis definitions Conference. Crit Care Med 2003;31:1250–6.
10. Rivers E, Nguyen B, Havstad S, et al. Early goal-directed therapy in the treatment of severe sepsis and septic shock. N Engl J Med 2001;345:1368–77.
11. Singer M, Deutschman CS, Seymour CW, et al. The third international consensus definitions for sepsis and septic shock (Sepsis-3). JAMA 2016;315(8):801–10.
12. Angus DC, Linde-Zwirble WT, Lidicker J, et al. Epidemiology of severe sepsis in the United States: analysis of incidence, outcome, and associated costs of care. Crit Care Med 2001;29:1303–10.
13. Kreitmann L, Monard C, Dauwalder O, et al. Early bacterial co-infection in ARDS related to COVID-19. Intensive Care Med 2020;46:1787–9.

14. Poston JT, Patel BK, Davis AM. Management of critically ill adults with COVID-19. JAMA 2020;323:1839–41.

15. Jui JEA. Ch. 146: septic shock. New York: McGraw-Hill; 2011.

16. CDC. "Sepsis Questions and Answers". 2014.

17. ellinger RPMC, Jean M, Masur H, et al. Surviving Sepsis Campaign guidelines for management of severe sepsis and septic shock. Crit Care Med 2004;32:858–73.

18. Liu VX, Fielding-Singh V, Greene JD, et al. The timing of early antibiotics and hospital mortality in sepsis. Am J Respir Crit Care Med 2017;196:856–63.

19. Aitken L, Williams G, Harvey M, et al. Nursing considerations to complement the surviving sepsis campaign guidelines. Crit Care Med 2011;39:1800–18.

20. Meddeb B, Hajjej Z, Gharsallah H, et al. Relationship between macrocirculation and microcirculation monitored by microdialysis during septic shock. Intensive Care Med Exp 2015;3:A522.

21. Romero-Brufau S, Gaines K, Nicolas CT, et al. The fifth vital sign? Nurse worry predicts inpatient deterioration within 24 hours. JAMIA Open 2019;2:465–70.

22. Saria S, Henry KE. Too many definitions of sepsis: can machine learning leverage the electronic health record to increase accuracy and bring consensus? Crit Care Med 2020;48:137–41.

23. Kleinpell R, Aitken L, Schorr CA. Implications of the new international sepsis guidelines for nursing care. Am J Crit Care 2013;22:212–22.

24. Gauer RL. Early recognition and management of sepsis in adults: the first six hours. Am Fam Physician 2013;1:44–53.

25. Alhazzani W, Møller MH, Arabi YM, et al. Surviving sepsis campaign: guidelines on the management of critically ill adults with coronavirus disease 2019. COVID 2020;48:e440–69.

26. Pickens CI, Wunderink RG. Principles and practice of antibiotic stewardship in the ICU. Chest 2019;156:163–71.

27. Seymour CW, Gesten F, Prescott HC, et al. Time to treatment and mortality during mandated emergency care for sepsis. N Engl J Med 2017;376:2235–44.

28. Reinhart K, Daniels R, Kissoon N, et al. Recognizing sepsis as a global health Priority — A WHO Resolution. N Engl J Med 2017;377:414–7.

Nursing Care for the Initial Resuscitation of Burn Patients

Mary G. Carey, PhD, RN[a],*,
Emily Katherine Valcin, DNP, RN, CNL, CCRN-K[b],
David Lent, DNP, MS, RN, CNL, CCRN-K, PCCN-K[c],
Mackenzie White, MS, RN[d]

KEYWORDS

- Burn resuscitation • Nursing care • Hospitalization • Critical care

KEY POINTS

- Nurses play an important role in the care of the initial resuscitation of burn patients.
- Over resuscitation, nicknamed "fluid creep," is one of the most important complications because it causes fluid overload in the following compartments: orbital, extremities, pulmonary, and abdominal, which are all associated with higher mortality.
- From the moment of the initial burn injury through treatment, rehabilitation, and beyond, pain control is a major nursing priority and challenge in the management of patients with burn injury.

INTRODUCTION

Burn injuries are very serious and are associated with substantial morbidity and mortality (**Fig. 1**). Burn injuries, particularly severe burn injuries, are accompanied by powerful immune and inflammatory responses, metabolic changes, and distributive shock that can lead to multiple organ failure and death. Nurses caring for patients with burn injuries are faced with a multitude of challenges to effectively manage care for these patients, including acute critical care management, rehabilitation, and long-term care.[1] Importantly, pain management must be a primary nursing consideration of burn care because it supports better wound management, sleep, participation in activities of daily living, quality of life, and long-term recovery.[2,3]

The American Burn Association (ABA) monitors and reports hospital admissions associated with specialized services provided by US burn centers. Demographically,

[a] Clinical Nursing Research Center, University of Rochester Medical Center, 601 Elmwood Avenue, Rochester, NY 14642, USA; [b] University of Rochester Medical Center, 601 Elmwood Avenue, Rochester, NY 14642, USA; [c] Adult Critical Care Outcomes, University of Rochester Medical Center, 601 Elmwood Avenue, Rochester, NY 14642, USA; [d] Burn/Trauma ICU, Adult Critical Care, University of Rochester Medical Center, 601 Elmwood Avenue, Rochester, NY 14642, USA
* Corresponding author.
E-mail address: Mary_Carey@URMC.Rochester.edu

Crit Care Nurs Clin N Am 33 (2021) 275–285
https://doi.org/10.1016/j.cnc.2021.05.004
0899-5885/21/© 2021 Elsevier Inc. All rights reserved.

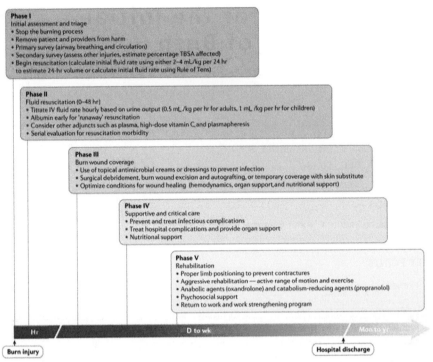

Fig. 1. The phases of burn care. (From Jeschke MG, van Baar ME, Choudhry MA, Chung KK, Gibran NS and Logsetty S. Burn injury. *Nat Rev Dis Primers.* 2020;6:11-11; with permission)

the distribution of burn patients is reported to be primarily men and boys (68%), and more than 40% of those occur among non-white patients. According to the ABA, causes of burn injuries include fire/flames (43%), scalding (34%), contact (9%), chemical (7%), and electrical (3%).[4] Environments that burn injuries occur varies, most commonly at home (78%), recreational environments (9%), followed by occupational environments (8%), and vehicular environments (5%). Although the overall survival rate is nearly 97%, those with burns greater than 25% of total body surface area (TBSA) are at risk of dying from smoke inhalation and other complications associated with burns.[4] Burns are the third leading cause of death in children under age 14 and are in the top 10 causes of death for all age groups. The young and the elderly are particularly vulnerable to local and systemic effects of burns because their skin is naturally thinner. In the United States, there are approximately 130 burn centers that admit more than 200 patients annually with burn injuries; the other 4500 acute care hospitals average fewer than 3 burn admissions per year. Thus, it is fair to conclude that first responders are appropriately diverting burn patients to dedicated burn centers.[5]

PHYSIOLOGY AND PATHOPHYSIOLOGY
Skin as an Organ

The skin is the largest organ of the body. Its multilayer design protects and regulates functions to help reduce water loss, contributes to innate and adaptive immunity, and is key in thermoregulation and sensory perception. In addition, skin also synthesizes vitamin D and contributes to bone formation, calcium metabolism, and immune regulation. The skin has 3 layers:

- Epidermis: The outermost and protective layer of skin that provides the critical waterproofing barrier, skin tone color, and continuously renews itself by shedding cells.
- Dermis: The middle layer that lies beneath the epidermis and senses touch and pain. It contains connective tissue, hair follicles, and sweat glands, fights infection, and has blood vessels for temperature regulation.
- Hypodermis: The deeper subcutaneous tissue composed of connective and adipose tissue that protects the muscle and bone from injury.

Pathophysiology of Burn Injuries

As with other organs, injuries to the skin are serious, and burn injuries especially so. A burn injury occurs when there is a disruption or death in some or all of the tissue cells, and severity is classified by the depth and zone of the affected tissue.[6] Burn injury to the skin may occur because of thermal or chemical source, radiation, electricity, friction, or another acute trauma.[6] Several factors influence the severity of the injury, and these are largely proportional to the magnitude and depth of the resulting tissue damage. Thermal burns are related to the duration of contact; that is, pH concentration in the case of chemical burns, or in the amount of current flow and resistance in case of an electrical burn. Similarly, the location of the burn plays a significant role in the physiologic response. The zone and depth of the burn disrupt the normal functions of the body that can result in shock, hypermetabolism, and immune dysregulation as the body naturally reacts to the insult. Inhalation burn injuries are especially serious and can result in life-threatening complications when lung tissue becomes significantly inflamed or is destroyed as a result of burn. Pulmonary complications, including pneumonia, increase mortality by 20%, and the diagnosis, via bronchoscopy and treatment, for example, beta-agonists, and so forth, remains under investigation; thus, the general clinical approach to inhalation injury is supportive care.[7]

THE 3 PHASES OF BURN CARE

Burns are classified according to the depth of tissue destruction, as superficial partial thickness, deep partial thickness, or full-thickness injuries (**Table 1**); importantly, burn wounds can have multiple stages of burns within the same wound. Acute care for severe burns can be compartmentalized into 3 distinct phases that overlap during the first days to weeks after initial burn injury: emergent, acute, and rehabilitative[1] (**Table 2**). The immediate postburn phase focuses on stopping the burning process because tissue destruction can extend hours after the burn occurred. The initial TBSA estimate is conducted, which helps to guide care during subsequent phases. The acute phase focuses primarily on fluid restoration in order to address hypovolemia that occurs as a result of fluid shifts, in order to preserve end-organ perfusion. In the rehabilitative phase, the focus shifts to controlling the body's metabolic response to the burn. In this phase, the wound may be surgically debrided and covered with a graft to promote rapid healing and to reduce infection risk. Supportive care and rehabilitation activities are prioritized, including physical and mental health support to enable the patient in returning to regular life.[1]

Phase I: Emergent

The emergent-resuscitative phase lasts from 48 to 72 hours after injury or until diuresis takes place. Because this phase is emergent, many interventions occur simultaneous to one another. Life-sustaining measures to manage airway, breathing, and circulation are accompanied by aggressive pain management and an estimation of TBSA effected by the burn. Burn centers use different methods to calculate TBSA. Some

Table 1
Classifications of burn injury

Name	Depth	Involvement	Consequences
First degree	Superficial partial thickness	The epidermis is injured or destroyed, and the dermis may also be involved	Painful but does not blister or scar
Second degree	Deep partial thickness	Involves the destruction of the epidermis and upper layers of the dermis and injury to the deeper portions of the dermis	Blisters and weeps With increasing depth, increased risk of infection With increasing depth, increased risk of scarring
Third degree	Full thickness	Involves total destruction of the epidermis and dermis, and in some cases, the destruction of the underlying tissue, muscle, and bone	Dry Insensate to light touch or pin prick Small areas will heal with substantial scar or contracture Large areas require skin grafting High risk of infection
Fourth degree	Full thickness	Involves muscle and bones	Loss of involved limb

Data from Jeschke MG, van Baar ME, Choudhry MA, Chung KK, Gibran NS and Logsetty S. Burn injury. *Nat Rev Dis Primers*. 2020;6:11-11.

use the "Rule of Nines," whereby different sections of the body are a multiple of 9, that is, each arm is 9%, each leg is 18%, circumferentially.[8] Using this method, patches of burned tissue that are not clearly delineated can be estimated by using the size of the patient's palm to be equivalent to 1%. Another method used is the Lund and Browder

Table 2
Nursing interventions for the phases of burn care

Emergent	Acute Phase	Rehabilitation
Promoting gas exchange and airway clearance	Restoring fluids and electrolyte balance	Promoting activity tolerance
Restoring fluids and electrolyte balance	Preventing infections	Improving body image and self-concept
Maintaining normal body temp	Monitoring cultures and white blood cells counts	Monitoring and managing complications
Minimizing pain and anxiety	Maintaining adequate nutrition	Teaching self-care
	Promoting skin integrity	
	Relieving pain and discomfort	
	Promoting physical mobility	
	Strengthen coping strategies	
	Supporting families	
	Monitoring and managing complications	

Data from Jeschke MG, van Baar ME, Choudhry MA, Chung KK, Gibran NS and Logsetty S. Burn injury. *Nat Rev Dis Primers*. 2020;6:11-11.

method, which also accounts for age.[9] As an outcome determinate, age, that is, both young and elderly, is strongly inversely correlated with survival.[10] Notably, the elderly are one of the fastest growing demographic of burn victims; thus, special attention is needed to optimize their survival and recovery.[10] It is also important to remember that when caring for a pediatric patient, their proportions must be accounted for when determining what percent of their skin is injured.

After the TBSA has been estimated, wounds are cleansed with chlorhexidine gluconate, and care consists of silver sulfadiazine or mafenide or bacitracin with wound care and surgical management as needed. To further prevent infection, continued care includes mechanical debridement by washing the surface of the wounds with mild soap or aseptic solutions. Then, the devitalized tissue is debrided, and often the wound is covered with antibacterial agents, such as silver sulfadiazine or bacitracin and occlusive dry cotton gauze.

Phase II: Acute

Fluid resuscitation

There are several fluid resuscitation formulas used to determine the total amount of fluids burn patients must receive within the first 24 hours of burn resuscitation as well as the rate of administration. The formula used varies depending on the burn center and based on what protocols they develop, but the ABA recommends lactated Ringer (LR) as a first-line choice because LR is the intravenous (IV) fluid that best mimics the fluid lost in a burn injury. If LR is not available, 0.9% sodium chloride (saline) solution is sufficient, but as soon as LR is available, it should replace the saline solution. In addition, if traditional LR is inadequate, some burn centers add albumin because albumin infusions optimize intravascular volume, which stabilizes the patient's hemodynamics during burn resuscitation.[11] Volume replacement is calculated based on the amount of fluid per kilogram of the patient's weight, per TBSA (%). Rates are continuously adjusted to maintain adequate urine output, which is closely monitored and used to approximate perfusion of end organs.

Importantly, during this phase of burn care, there is the risk of both underresuscitation and overresuscitation. Fortunately, underresuscitation is uncommon given the adherence to weight and injury-based formulas. Overresuscitation, nicknamed "fluid creep," is one of the most important complications because it causes fluid overload in the following compartments: orbital, extremities, pulmonary, and abdominal, which are all associated with higher mortality.[12]

Hypothermia

Patients with large burns often present in the Emergency Department with hypothermia after suffering a thermal burn because of exposure during and immediately after the accident, cooling of the burn wound, and time to hospital transfer. In a recent study, the medical records of patients (n = 57) with thermal burns affecting more than 15% of body surface area indicated that 80% developed hypothermia on admission. They presented with burns more than 35% $\pm$ 17% of their body surface, with 28% $\pm$ 18% being deep burns. Mortality during the hospitalizations was high, nearly 30%. Thus, the presence of hypothermia during the acute phase was statistically related to death ($P = .033$), and it was observed that hypothermia is directly related to the extent of the burn ($P = .003$).[13] A priority for nursing care is rapidly reheating to avoid this heat loss; thus, nurses must know and promptly administer adequate reheating measures to improve chances of survival in major burns. Such measures include using a precision temperature management system, which provides rapid patient warming with accuracy to optimize patient outcomes, for example, fluid warmers and forced-air blanket warmers.

Burn wound coverage

Early excision of necrotic tissue and closure of the burn wound have been major advancements in treating human patients with severe thermal injuries in the past 20 years.[14] The acute-wound coverage phase, which varies depending on the extent of injury, lasts until the wounds have been covered, either through the normal healing process or through grafting. Risk for infection is high during this phase, so careful monitoring of wounds, surveillance of blood cultures, and administration of prophylactic antibiotics are necessary.

Grafting is an important burn treatment therapy used to reduce the body's systemic hypermetabolic response to the injury and promote more rapid healing. Grafting is accomplished by excising viable tissue from areas at a depth and size proportional to the injury. In both minor and major burns, grafting helps to reduce the risk of wound infection, can diminish contractures, and may also improve both functional and cosmetic outcomes for the patient.[6] There are numerous types of skin grafts, including autograft (obtained from patient's own donor site), allograft (obtained from another person), xenograft (obtained from another species), homograft (donated cadaver skin), and synthetic skin products. In the case of autologous grafts, they are harvested from the patient in either single- or multistage surgeries and are covered with nonadherent dressings to avoid dislodgement of the graft through mechanical shearing force. Regardless of type, all grafts should be carefully monitored for tissue adherence and revascularization.[6]

Phase III: Rehabilitation

This important phase includes care and closure of the wound, prevention, and treatment of complications, including infection. As the burn injury continues to heal, resolution of the wound results in scar formation with a gradual return to normal tissue function by focusing on critical aspects of supportive care. Optimizing nutritional support to improve wound healing is an essential nursing responsibility during this phase given the high metabolic demands of wound healing; many patients require enteral feedings and/or protein and caloric supplementation.[15] Inpatient rehabilitation takes place during the convalescent-rehabilitative phase. Although principles of rehabilitation are included in the plan of care from the day of admission, during this time, home exercises and wound care are taught to the patient and family. Wound management includes maintenance and assessment of surgically grafted skin, or placement of synthetic membranes. In addition, pressure appliances to reduce scarring or braces to prevent contractures are fitted to the patient.

Rehabilitation planning must start from the time of injury. Having a substantial burn injury is frightening, particularly as patients will not know what to expect and will often be in pain. Consistent and often repetitive education is a vital part of patient care. Nursing care initiates and focuses on edema management, respiratory management, positioning, and engaging patients in functional activities and movement. During this phase, adequate pain control is crucially important to achieve desired outcomes and preburn movement habits. In recent years, burn care has improved so much that survival expectations are often met, and there is a larger focus on quality of life for burn survivors, including mobility, form, function, and physical appearance.

SPECIAL CONSIDERATION FOR NURSING CARE IN THE RESUSCITATION OF BURN PATIENTS

The Psychology of Burns

Of significant importance is that the injury not only affects the physical health but also may have substantial long-term implications for the mental health and quality of life of the patient. Accordingly, patients with burn injury cannot be considered recovered when the burn wounds have healed; instead, burn injury leads to long-term profound alterations that must be addressed to optimize quality of life. Research has demonstrated that even 2 years after a burn injury, patients who experienced high levels of pain during the acute period develop long-term sequalae and suffer with acute distress disorder, depression, suicide, posttraumatic stress disorder, or other negative long-term psychological effects.[16]

Diagnostic Tests for Burn Care

Routine tests conducted on patients admitted with burn injuries include complete blood count, complete metabolic panel, urinalysis, chest X ray, and similar tests. These tests provide early assessment of hemodynamic changes, that is, anemia as well as changes in renal function. The chest X ray reveals inhalation injury, the development of a pneumonia, changes associated with acute respiratory distress syndrome, and so forth. The complete metabolic serum panel provides information on electrolyte status, guiding the type of IV fluid to use, monitoring renal function, as well as whether additional electrolytes are needed.

Pharmacologic Drugs for Burn Care

A patient with burn injuries is particularly vulnerable to infection because they have lost the first line of defense, the skin. In fact, postburn infection is a major cause of morbidity and mortality; therefore, it is helpful to review topical antibiotics used to treat those with burns. Other complications of burns include anemia and stress ulcers. A review of medications used to treat anemia as well as medications to prevent ulcers and the bleeding that can occur would be helpful. Narcotic analgesics, particularly opiate derivatives, are often used in controlling pain and providing sedation during the emergent and intermediate phases of burn care. The use of an adjunct bowel regimen is important while patients are on narcotic analgesics to ensure the prevention of obstruction or ileus. The most common pharmacologic drugs used with burn care include topical antibiotics; antiemetic; antacids; narcotic analgesics; and anxiolytics. Overall, it is important for nurses to be familiar with the common problems associated with burns that require pharmacologic management (**Table 3**).

Table 3 Pharmacologic management of burn injuries	
Condition	**Pharmacologic Options**
Pain	Nonopioid analgesics Anxiolytics Anesthetics Opioid analgesics
Anxiety	Benzodaiepines SSRI antidepressants Buspirone (BuSpar)
Pruritus	Eutectic Mixture of Local Anesthetics Topical doxepin Vaseline-based creams Cocoa butter Mineral oil Hydrogel sheets Topical glucocorticoids

From Demling RH. Burns: what are the pharmacologic treatment options? *Expert Opin Pharmacother.* 2008;9:1895-908

Pain Management for Burn Care

Despite profound improvements in modern burn care, suboptimal and inconsistent pain management may persist throughout all stages of burn treatment. Without aggressive pain control throughout recovery, patients are likely to suffer not only from the acute pain of the injury but also from secondary morbidities, including long-term anxiety and posttraumatic stress, and potentially delayed wound healing. Burn pain is further complicated by a relative lack of standardized approaches across burn centers. Instead of applying evidence-based care, variability exists within pain management strategies that may affect the overall recovery for the patient. The complex interaction of anatomic, physiologic, pharmacologic, psychosocial, and premorbid issues can make the treatment of burn pain particularly difficult, and it is important to avoid undertreatment.[17]

From the moment of the initial burn injury through treatment, rehabilitation, and beyond, pain control is a major nursing priority and challenge in the management of patients with burn injury. In fact, evidence suggests that burn pain is among the most difficult to treat among any cause of acute pain.[18] The aim of analgesic drugs should be to develop baseline pain control to allow functional movement and activities of daily living to occur at any time during the day. In addition to the actual burn injury, the therapies used to treat burn injuries exacerbate the difficulty of pain control because most of these interventions are associated with pain, including dressing changes, excision and grafting, and physical therapy. Ironically, these restorative therapies can cause pain that is equivalent to or worse than the pain of an initial burn injury. Therefore, pain management must be a foundational consideration of burn care for nursing.

CASE STUDY

A 24-year-old victim was rescued from an apartment fire in which they suffered severe burns to face and body; soot was found on their face and in the nose. Upon initial assessment, course lung sounds were auscultated, and the individual was immediately placed on 100% Fio_2 nonrebreather by first responders and warmed during transport. Upon arrival to the regional burn center, the victim was subsequently intubated to protect their airway. The patient suffered 51% burns of their TBSA; specifically, circumferential burns to bilateral arms, burns to face, abdomen, back, buttocks, and legs.

Day 1

Vital Signs	ABGs	Laboratory Tests	Therapies
T-Max 38	pH 7.30	BG 92	• Intubation for airway protection
HR 161	Pao_2 80	Hb 17	• Rewarming
BP 83/55	$Paco_2$ 36.8	HCT 44	• Bronchoscopy with bronchioloalveolar lavage
UOP 5 cc/h	HCO 17	Na 130	• Administer humidified o_2
	BE 8.0	Cl 104	• Central access achieved
		K+ 4.9	• Fluid resuscitation for evaporative loss (1 mL × kg × %TBSA)/24 h
			• UOP goal 40 mL/h
			• Aggressive pain control
			• Rewarming
			• Wound management/dressing
			• Albumin administration
			• High-calorie, high-protein via naso-duodenal feeding tube
			• Every 1 hour Doppler signal checks of wounds and grafts

Day 2

Vital Signs	ABGs	Laboratory Tests	Therapies
BP 108/68	pH 7.35	BG 88	• Second bronchoscopy with bronchioalveolar lavage
UOP 26 cc/h	Pao$_2$ 88	Hb 15	• Aggressive wound care and pain management
	Paco$_2$ 38	HCT 40	• Rewarming
	HCO 20	Na 135	• Wound management/dressing
	BE 8.0	Cl 103	• Fluid resuscitation
		K+ 4.4	• High-protein nutritional support

Day 3 to 8

Vital Signs	ABGs	Laboratory Tests	Therapies
WNL	pH 7.41	WNL	• IV sedation off
Goal UOP met >40 cc/h	Pao$_2$ 92		• Transition to enteral pain control
	Paco$_2$ 39		• PRN IV pain medication PRN for wound care
	HCO 20		• Continue high-calorie, high-protein diet
	BE 8.0		• Foley irrigation, Zosyn, ceftriaxone
			• Physical and occupational therapy consult
			• OOB to chair with goal to ambulate on ventilator 100 feet by day 4 progressing to 300 feet by day 8

Day 9: Discharge to home

Vital Signs	ABGs	Laboratory Tests	Therapies
WNL	WNL	WNL	• Extubate to high-flow humidified nasal cannula
UOP >30 cc/h			• PRN pain and anxiety medication
			• Increased ambulation focus on range of motion restoration as tolerated

Abbreviations: ABG, arterial blood gas; BE, base excess; BG, blood glucose; BP, blood pressure; Cl, chloride; Hb, hemoglobin; HCO, bicarbonate; HCT, hematocrit; HR, heart rate; K+, potassium; Na, sodium; OOB, out of bed; Pao$_2$, partial pressure of oxygen; Paco$_2$, partial pressure of carbon dioxide; UOP, urine output; PRN, as needed; T-Max, maximum temperature; WNL, within normal limits.

Case Study Clinical Questions

1. Which laboratory result would be expected during the emergent phase of a burn injury?
   A. Glucose 100 mg/dL
   B. Potassium 3.5 mEq/L
   C. Sodium 142 mEq/L
   D. Albumin 4.2 g/dL
2. On the third postburn day, the nurse finds that the patient's hourly urine output is 26 mL. The nurse should continue to assess and notify the provider for an order to:
   A. Decrease the rate of the intravenous infusion
   B. Change the type of intravenous fluid being administered

C. Change the urinary catheter

D. Increase the rate of the intravenous infusion

3. A Jewish patient requires grafting to promote burn healing. Which graft is most likely to be unacceptable to the patient?

A. Isograft

B. Autograft

C. Homograft

D. Xenograft

Case Study Answers

1. Answer A is correct. During the emergent phase, glucose levels increase as a result of the stress response.

    Answers B, C, and D are within normal range. K+ and Na+ would be observed to be elevated, whereas albumin would be lowered during the emergent period because of increased cell permeability.

2. Answer D is correct. Urinary output should be maintained between 30 mL and 50 mL per hour. The first action taken should be to increase the IV rate of isotonic fluids to prevent increased acidosis.

    Answer A would lead to diminished output, so it is incorrect. Answer B is incorrect; there is no indication that the type of IV fluid is not appropriate. Answer C would not increase the patient's urine output and would place the patient at greater risk for infection.

3. Answer D is correct. Xenografts are taken from nonhuman sources. The most common sources are porcine, or pigskin, which would be offensive to those of both Jewish and Muslim faith.

    Answer A refers to a graft taken from an identical twin. Answer B is incorrect because it refers to a graft taken from the patient's own skin. Answer C refers to a graft taken from a cadaver.

DISCUSSION

As this case study illustrates, optimal care for the severe burn patient is time critical and resource intensive. To achieve optimal outcomes, burn centers should be staffed by highly trained nurses, familiar with the modalities of care and the recovery trajectory of the patient. Nurse-driven care should meld seamlessly as part of an interdisciplinary, coordinated effort to restore the patient to the highest level of functioning possible. Importantly, there is the risk of underresuscitation and overresuscitation; both are undesirable, and if the patient is admitted to a burn center, these complications are very unusual.[12]

SUMMARY

Burn injuries are serious and account for about 2 million injuries each year in the United States. According to the ABA (2016), more than 50,000 persons require hospitalization each year for burn care and rehabilitation.[5]

CLINICS CARE POINTS

- Successful burn care requires focused efforts from a team of experienced health care workers committed to treating the patient through the continuum of acute burn care and rehabilitation.

- Without aggressive pain control throughout recovery, patients are likely to suffer not only from the acute pain of the injury but also from secondary morbidities, including long-term anxiety and posttraumatic stress, and potentially delayed wound healing.
- In recent years, burn care has improved so much that survival expectations are often met and there is a larger focus on quality of life for burn survivors, including mobility, form, function, and physical appearance.

DISCLOSURE

The authors have nothing to disclose.

REFERENCES

1. Jeschke MG, van Baar ME, Choudhry MA, et al. Burn injury. Nat Rev Dis Primers 2020;6:11.
2. Raymond I, Ancoli-Israel S, Choinière M. Sleep disturbances, pain and analgesia in adults hospitalized for burn injuries. Sleep Med 2004;5:551–9.
3. Christian LM, Graham JE, Padgett DA, et al. Stress and wound healing. Neuroimmunomodulation 2006;13:337–46.
4. Association AB. Burn injury fact sheet. Chicago, IL: American Burn Association; 2018.
5. Association AB. Burn incidence fact sheet. Chicago, IL: American Burn Association; 2016.
6. Kagan RJ, Peck MD, Ahrenholz DH, et al. Surgical management of the burn wound and use of skin substitutes: an expert panel white paper. J Burn Care Res 2013;34:e60–79.
7. Dries DJ, Endorf FW. Inhalation injury: epidemiology, pathology, treatment strategies. Scand J Trauma Resusc Emerg Med 2013;21:31.
8. Moore RA, Waheed A, Burns B. Rule of Nines. In: StatPearls. Treasure Island, FL: StatPearls Publishing Copyright © 2020, StatPearls Publishing LLC; 2020.
9. Godwin Z, Tan J, Bockhold J, et al. Development and evaluation of a novel smart device-based application for burn assessment and management. Burns 2015;41:754–60.
10. Jeschke MG, Pinto R, Costford SR, et al. Threshold age and burn size associated with poor outcomes in the elderly after burn injury. Burns 2016;42:276–81.
11. Bedi MK, Sarabahi S, Agrawal K. New fluid therapy protocol in acute burn from a tertiary burn care centre. Burns 2019;45:335–40.
12. Bacomo FK, Chung KK. A primer on burn resuscitation. J Emerg Trauma Shock 2011;4:109–13.
13. Alonso-Fernández JM, Lorente-González P, Pérez-Munguía L, et al. Analysis of hypothermia through the acute phase in major burns patients: nursing care. Enferm Intensiva 2020;31:120–30.
14. Gomez M, Wong DT, Stewart TE, et al. The FLAMES score accurately predicts mortality risk in burn patients. J Trauma 2008;65:636–45.
15. Moreira E, Burghi G, Manzanares W. Update on metabolism and nutrition therapy in critically ill burn patients. Med Intensiva 2018;42:306–16.
16. Young AW, Dewey WS, King BT. Rehabilitation of burn injuries: an update. Phys Med Rehabil Clin N Am 2019;30:111–32.
17. Griggs C, Goverman J, Bittner EA, et al. Sedation and pain management in burn patients. Clin Plast Surg 2017;44:535–40.
18. Patterson DR, Hoflund H, Espey K, et al. Pain management. Burns 2004;30:A10–5.

Pediatric Resuscitation

Amanda P. Bettencourt, PhD, APRN, CCRN-K, ACCNS-P[a],*,
Melissa Gorman, MSN, RN, NPD-BC, CCRN-K[b],
Jodi E. Mullen, MS, RN-BC, CCRN, CCNS, ACCNS-P, FCCM[c]

KEYWORDS

- Pediatric resuscitation • Cardiac arrest • Postresuscitation care • Family presence
- Pediatric advanced life support

KEY POINTS

- The cause of pediatric cardiopulmonary arrest differs in etiology and pathophysiology from those of adults.
- Early detection of clinical decompensation can prevent most cases of pediatric cardiopulmonary arrest in children.
- Pediatric resuscitation management should follow the American Heart Association Pediatric Advanced Life Support Recommendations.
- Postresuscitation nursing care includes monitoring oxygenation and ventilation, supporting hemodynamics, temperature and seizure control, and managing electrolytes.
- Outcomes after cardiopulmonary arrest can be optimized by a clinician training regimen that includes basic and advanced life support skills, behavioral skills to enhance leadership and communication, and the use of high-fidelity clinical simulation training.

INTRODUCTION

The etiology, pathophysiology, and outcomes from pediatric cardiopulmonary arrest are distinct from those seen in adults.[1] Cardiac arrest occurs much less frequently in children than in adults. Although survival has improved dramatically over the past 20 to 30 years, several key factors such as prompt recognition, adherence to pediatric-specific resuscitation guidelines, and high-quality postresuscitation care and monitoring affect the likelihood of a good quality of life after an arrest.[1] A critical intervention in pediatric nursing is recognizing the precipitating factors for cardiac arrest and intervening early to prevent it. If an arrest does occur, the child's survival and an excellent postarrest outcome are linked to nurses' expert performance of pediatric-

Funded by: NHLBI. Grant number(s): K12HL13803.
[a] Department of Systems, Populations, and Leadership, University of Michigan School of Nursing, 400 North Ingalls Building, Room #4304, Ann Arbor, MI 48109-5482, USA; [b] Shriners Hospitals for Children-Boston, 51 Blossom Street, Boston, MA 02114, USA; [c] Pediatric Intensive Care Unit, UF Health Shands Children's Hospital, 1600 SW Archer Rd., Gainesville FL 32608, USA
* Corresponding author.
E-mail address: abetten@med.umich.edu

Crit Care Nurs Clin N Am 33 (2021) 287–302
https://doi.org/10.1016/j.cnc.2021.05.005
0899-5885/21/© 2021 Elsevier Inc. All rights reserved.

specific resuscitation interventions. The purpose of this article is to promote excellence in nurses' early detection of deterioration, outline the latest evidence-based pediatric resuscitation nursing interventions, and describe the process of expert post-arrest nursing care that ensures the best possible patient outcome.

DISCUSSION
Detecting Decompensation in Children

A review of the data across a pediatric safety collaborative suggests that 16% of in-hospital pediatric resuscitations are a result of failing to detect decompensation in a timely fashion and escalate care.[2] Detecting decompensation early in children is difficult because children are often unable or willing to report their symptoms. Their physiology allows for a prolonged period of stable decompensation before a rapid decline occurs. Nurses are the primary providers of ongoing patient surveillance. Nurses collect subjective and objective assessment data, interpret and synthesize that data, and then determine potential interventions and threats to their patients' health and safety. Therefore, it is not surprising that efforts to detect decompensation in children as early as possible focus on nursing surveillance and assessment.

Table 1 lists the typical clinical manifestations of decompensation found in children. Standardized early warning triggers and tools, such as the Pediatric Early Warning Score (PEWS) and its variants,[3] and the Rothman Index (RI)[4] or other prediction algorithms exist to assist nurses and other caregivers in identifying patients who are beginning to show signs of decompensation. The components of these standard tools are also noted in **Table 1**. While the PEWS requires an active assessment and input of a score by the nurse and the RI uses nursing data entered into the electronic medical record to generate its score, the goal of both tools is to translate subjective and objective nursing assessment data into a number that is meaningful to the care team and inspires action.

A recent systematic review of the validity and effectiveness of the plethora of early warning systems and trigger tools suggests in general that they are very good at predicting transfers of patients to the intensive care unit, but that they often overestimate the child's decompensation, which may lead to inappropriate transfers and alarm fatigue.[5] Another potential issue with scoring tools is that nurses do not score the same patient the same way consistently.[5] Most studies of the ability of these tools to effectively decrease mortality or cardiorespiratory arrest events have methodologic concerns, which limit their ability to demonstrate benefit.[5] Evidence does suggest that these triggers and tools are appropriate and evidence-based additions to a comprehensive nursing surveillance plan that focuses on identifying the signs and symptoms of clinical decompensation in children as early as possible.

Identification of Acute Decompensation

Assessment principles
Timely recognition and response to pediatric decompensation is vital to improve cardiac arrest outcomes. A standardized approach to rapid assessment and intervention is an essential component of most formal life support courses such as the American Heart Association (AHA) Pediatric Advanced Life Support (PALS). Throughout the assessment process, when a life-threatening problem is identified, appropriate interventions are initiated immediately. The first step in this standardized approach is a general observational assessment. The Pediatric Assessment Triangle (PAT) is a tool that was designed to standardize the rapid evaluation of infants and children for all levels of health-care providers. It helps to establish the level of severity and

Table 1
Clinical signs of decompensation and early warning/trigger tools

System	Sign	Early vs. Late Sign	Included in Tool or Trigger System
Neurologic	Change in the level of consciousness/behavior	Early	PEWS Rothman Index
	Fever/temperature	Early	PEWS Rothman Index
	Pain	Late	PEWS
Respiratory	Respiratory rate	Late	PEWS Rothman Index
	Work of breathing	Early	Rothman Index
	Oxygen saturation	Late	PEWS Rothman Index
	Receiving oxygen therapy	Late	PEWS Rothman Index
	Airway clearance problems	Early	PEWS Rothman Index
	Laboratory results	Early	Rothman Index
Cardiac	Systolic blood pressure	Late	PEWS Rothman Index
	Pulses	Early	PEWS Rothman Index
	Capillary refill time	Early	PEWS Rothman Index
	ECG rhythm	Late	Rothman Index
	Laboratory results	Late	Rothman Index
Integumentary	Skin color	Early	PEWS Rothman Index
Other Subjective Assessments	Staff concern	Early	PEWS
	Family concern	Early	PEWS

The PEWS denotes the original PEWS and its validated variants, such as the CHEWS, CCHEWS, and so forth.
Abbreviation: CCHEWS, Cardiac Children's Hospital Early Warning Score; CHEWS, Children's Hospital Early Warning Score; ECG, electrocardiogram.

prioritize the treatment needed. The PAT consists of three components: appearance, work of breathing, and circulation of the skin.[6] A primary assessment, including vital signs, should follow the PAT. The primary assessment is a hands-on evaluation that focuses on the airway, breathing, circulation, disability, and exposure. The secondary assessment is performed next, including a focused history and detailed physical examination with ongoing reassessment.[7] **Table 2** presents a summary of the key clinical assessment findings in acute pediatric decompensation.

Management principles
Pediatric resuscitation management should follow evidence-based recommendations such as those outlined in the AHA PALS guidelines.[7] The AHA, in cooperation with the International Liaison Committee on Resuscitation, updates these guidelines based on a continuous evidence evaluation process and publishes focused updates.

High-quality cardiopulmonary resuscitation and rapid defibrillation
- High-quality cardiopulmonary resuscitation (CPR) is the cornerstone of pediatric resuscitation. Current AHA guidelines emphasize the importance of rapid recognition of cardiac arrest, immediate initiation of high-quality chest compressions,

Table 2	
Key clinical assessment findings for acute decompensation	

Respiratory Distress	• Increase in respiratory effort
	  ○ Tachypnea
	  ○ Accessory muscle use
	  ○ Retractions
	• Abnormal airway sounds
	  ○ Wheezing
	• Stridor
	• Change in the level of consciousness

Respiratory Failure	• Inadequate respiratory effort
	  ○ Apnea
	  ○ Bradypnea
	• Hypoxemia despite supplemental oxygen
	  ○ Cyanosis
	• Decreased level of consciousness
	• Bradycardia

Shock	• Signs of impaired perfusion
	  ○ Weak central pulses
	  ○ Diminished peripheral pulses
	  ○ Prolonged capillary refill
	  ○ Cool mottled skin
	• Hypotension
	• Tachycardia
	• Oliguria
	• Altered mental status

Cardiovascular Compromise or Cardiac Arrest	• Changes in heart rate or rhythm
	  ○ Tachycardia
	  ○ Bradycardia
	  ○ Arrhythmia
	  ○ Weak or absent pulse
	• Hypotension
	• Signs of shock
	• Decreased level of consciousness
	• Sudden collapse

and delivery of effective ventilations.[8] In pediatric patients, this involves compressions that are one-third the anterior-posterior depth of the chest, at a rate of 100 to 120 compressions per minute, and allow for good chest recoil.[8] When providing CPR without an advanced airway, the ratio of compressions to ventilations for pediatric patients is 30:2 when a single rescuer is present and 15:2 when multiple rescuers are present.[8] When performing CPR on infants and children with an advanced airway present, one breath should be delivered every 2 to 3 seconds while providing continuous compressions.[8] When providing respirations, clinicians must avoid excessive ventilation, and ventilation volume should produce no more than visible chest rise.[9]

○ Defibrillation: Clinicians must initiate rapid defibrillation for ventricular fibrillation and pulseless ventricular tachycardia (VF/pVT) without delay. The shorter the duration of VF/pVT, the more likely the shock will result in a perfusing rhythm.[8] Manual defibrillators are preferred to automated external defibrillators in infants and children because the energy dose can be titrated to the patient's weight.[8] In infants and children, the initial defibrillation dose is 2 J/kg and 4 to 10 J/kg for subsequent defibrillation attempts.[8]

○ Physiologic and quality monitoring during CPR: Although not required, when available, the team may use additional monitoring modalities to assess the quality of CPR. Arterial blood pressure monitoring may be beneficial for evaluating blood pressures achieved during resuscitation. End-tidal carbon dioxide monitoring may also indicate CPR's effectiveness and the return of spontaneous circulation (ROSC).[8] CPR feedback devices may also improve the quality of compressions performed.[8]

Airway

○ Respiratory distress: Prompt recognition and management of respiratory distress in children is essential because respiratory distress can lead to respiratory arrest, which, if left untreated, can lead to cardiac arrest. Interventions to manage respiratory distress include general principles to ensure a patent airway and deliver oxygen as needed. Nurses may accomplish this by repositioning, suctioning, or administering supplemental oxygen via a nasal cannula or face mask. When the cause of respiratory distress is identified (for example, asthma, pneumonia, or croup), children will require specific interventions based on the nature and severity of clinical symptoms.

○ Respiratory failure: Because most pediatric cardiac arrests are caused by respiratory failure, airway management is a resuscitation priority. This may be accomplished by bag mask ventilation (BMV) or placement of an advanced airway. When performed correctly, BMV may be as effective as ventilation through an advanced airway for short periods. During cardiac arrest, the benefits of an advanced airway include the ability to provide uninterrupted compressions, monitor CPR effectiveness/ROSC via end-tidal CO_2 monitoring, and decrease aspiration risk. However, placement of an advanced airway in a pediatric patient requires specialized equipment and training. A recent systematic review of the literature[10] concluded that there is insufficient evidence to suggest improved survival to hospital discharge after placement of an advanced airway (tracheal tube or supraglottic airway) during cardiac arrest in children. The current recommendation of the 2019 American Heart Association focused update on Pediatric Advanced Life Support states that BMV is reasonable compared with advanced airway interventions in managing children during cardiac arrest in the out-of-hospital setting.[11] No recommendation was made for or against the use of an advanced airway for in-hospital cardiac arrest (IHCA) management.[11] The recommendations also note that the team should consider transport time, providers' skill level, and equipment availability to select the most appropriate airway intervention. If BMV is ineffective despite proper techniques, more advanced airway interventions should be considered.[11]

Shock. Rapid identification and treatment of pediatric shock is a priority because untreated shock can progress to cardiac arrest. Shock is defined as a physiologic state characterized by inadequate tissue perfusion to meet metabolic demand and tissue oxygenation. Shock states can be classified by the type of shock, including hypovolemic, cardiogenic, distributive, and obstructive. The most common type of pediatric shock is hypovolemic, including shock due to bleeding.[8]

Hypovolemic shock occurs owing to decreased intravascular volume. This may be due to fluid losses from vomiting and diarrhea, burns, hemorrhage, or inadequate fluid intake. Cardiogenic shock is a result of myocardial dysfunction and may be caused by congenital heart disease, cardiomyopathy, myocarditis, or arrhythmia. Distributive shock occurs in states that result in decreased systemic vascular resistance that leads to inadequate blood flow. Septic shock, anaphylactic shock, and neurogenic shock are all examples of distributive shock. Obstructive shock refers to conditions that impair flow of blood to or from the heart, resulting in decreased cardiac output. Pericardial tamponade, tension pneumothorax, and pulmonary embolism are all examples of obstructive shock.[7] Multiple types of shock may co-occur,[8] and it is important to identify the type of shock to direct treatment.

The severity of shock may be categorized as hypotensive or compensated (normal systolic blood pressure with inadequate tissue perfusion). In children, compensatory mechanisms such as tachycardia and vasoconstriction are often present. As compensatory mechanisms fail, patients may develop hypotension, decreased mental status, and reduced urine output. Hypotension is a late sign of most types of shock and may indicate impending cardiac arrest.[7]

Treatment of shock includes supporting the airway, oxygenation, and ventilation, establishing vascular access, and providing fluid resuscitation while monitoring, reassessing, and providing medications as indicated to treat the underlying cause. Fluid resuscitation is a priority in treating most types of shock; however, clinicians must take caution to administer adequate volume while avoiding fluid overload. Generally, fluid resuscitation involves administering isotonic crystalloid as a 20 mL/kg bolus administered over 5 to 20 minutes.[7] Exceptions to this are 10 to 20 mL/kg for septic shock and 5 to 10 mL/kg over 10 to 20 minutes for cardiogenic shock.[7] Patients with signs of shock should be reassessed after each fluid bolus to assess fluid responsiveness and signs of volume overload.[8]

Management of cardiogenic shock differs from other types of shock. Rapid boluses or large volumes may worsen cardiac function and increase the risk of pulmonary edema. Cardiogenic shock is caused by myocardial dysfunction, so management should be directed at improving cardiac output by increasing the efficiency of ventricular ejection while minimizing myocardial demand.[7] Some children with cardiogenic shock have a high preload and do not require additional fluid administration, whereas others may require cautious fluid administration to optimize preload. Fluid administration may include smaller fluid boluses of 5 to 10 mL/kg administered over 10 to 20 minutes with close assessment and stopping the infusion if deterioration occurs. Afterload reduction is an effective way to increase stroke volume, but patients with hypotension may require fluid therapy and inotropic support to tolerate afterload reduction.[7] Vasodilators, inotropes, and inodilators may be administered in cardiogenic shock to reduce peripheral vascular resistance and/or improve contractility.[7] In a normotensive child in cardiogenic shock with evidence of pulmonary edema, diuretics may be indicated. A pediatric critical care or pediatric cardiology specialist should be consulted to guide therapy for cardiogenic shock.[7]

Additional treatment of shock states must be initiated based on the identified type of shock. The Surviving Sepsis Campaign International Guidelines for the Management of Septic Shock and Sepsis-Associated Organ Dysfunction in Children[12] outlines essential components for management of patients in septic shock. Key elements of these guidelines include prompt administration of antibiotics as soon as possible and within 1 hour of sepsis recognition and administration of vasoactive infusions in patients with signs of low perfusion despite fluid administration.[12]

Vascular access. During pediatric decompensation, vascular access is critical for administration of medications and intravenous fluids. Pediatric vascular access can be challenging, especially in the setting of cardiac arrest or altered perfusion. When the team cannot rapidly obtain intravenous access, intraosseous (IO) cannulation can be a safe and reliable vascular access method in children and infants. When placed correctly, IO catheters can administer intravenous (IV) fluids, blood products, and medications. In certain circumstances, such as cardiac arrest, IO may be the initial vascular access attempted.[7]

Estimating the patient's weight. In pediatric resuscitation, most medication doses and intravenous fluid volumes are weight based. A team member should record an accurate weight in kilograms in the patient's medical record.[13] Pediatric patients may present in settings wherein a precise weight is unknown or unable to be obtained. When an exact weight cannot be obtained using traditional methods, height-based weight estimation tools such as the Broselow pediatric emergency tape are often used. The Broselow pediatric emergency tape is a standardized tape that is placed flat next to the patient, with one end aligned to the top of the head. When positioned next to the patient, the area on the tape adjacent to the heel is used to determine an estimated weight of the patient based on the height. This card also includes color-coded emergency medication dosing and equipment sizing based on the height estimate. Code carts and equipment storage can also be organized based on this color-coded system. Benefits include the ability to use the tape without interruption of resuscitation efforts and ease of use. Potential disadvantages of this method include the inability to factor in body habitus, especially in the population of patients with obesity.[14]

Medications and supplies. A well-organized emergency supply cart with pediatric-specific equipment and medication dosing guides should be available in settings wherein pediatric patients are treated. Supplies must be available in sizes to accommodate pediatric patients treated in that area. Clinicians may use color-based coding systems to ensure proper equipment and correct medication dosing based on the patient's weight.[13]

During pediatric resuscitation, accurate drug administration is a critical skill that has the potential for error owing to high stress and the need for weight-based calculations in the pediatric population. Standardized concentrations and medication dosing systems that minimize calculations may reduce the likelihood of medication errors.[13] Comprehensive bedside medication dosing reference tools like those shown in **Figs. 1** and **2** containing information on drug dilution, preparation, and volume to administer are more likely to result in accurate drug administration.[15]

Drugs administered during pediatric resuscitation will vary depending on circumstances, but epinephrine and antiarrhythmics are often administered in cardiac arrest. Epinephrine is administered to optimize cardiac perfusion and restore spontaneous circulation during cardiac arrest.[8] Current recommendations state that it is reasonable to administer epinephrine every 3 to 5 minutes during cardiac arrest, with the initial dose being given within 5 minutes of the start of chest compressions.[8] For shock-refractory ventricular fibrillation or ventricular tachycardia, lidocaine or amiodarone may be administered.[8]

Team dynamics and communication. Pediatric resuscitation requires a multidisciplinary team of providers to work together to achieve optimal outcomes effectively. The team leader and all team members must establish clear roles and responsibilities, be aware of limitations, offer constructive interventions, and share information.[7] Communication techniques such as closed-loop communication, speaking clearly and calmly, and displaying mutual respect[7] must be demonstrated during pediatric resuscitation. One observational study by El-Shafy and colleagues[16] found that the use of closed-loop communication can increase the speed and efficiency of task completion in the pediatric trauma resuscitation setting. Resuscitation teams should

Weight (kg)			2 kg	3 kg	5 kg	7.5 kg	10 kg
Age			Premature	Newborn	1 mo	6 mo	1 yr
ET tube size			3.0–3.5	3.0–3.5	3.5	3.5–4.0	4.0
Adenosine	Conc = 3 mg/mL	Dose	0.1 mg/kg	0.15 mg	0.3 mg	0.6 mg	0.75 mg	0.9 mg
Administer by rapid IV/IO bolus		Volume	0.03 mL/kg	0.05 mL	0.1 mL	0.2 mL	0.25 mL	0.3 mL
Amiodarone	Conc = 50 mg/mL	Dose	5 mg/kg	10 mg	15 mg	25 mg	37.5 mg	50 mg
Administer IV/IO		Volume	0.1 mL/kg	0.2 mL	0.3 mL	0.5 mL	0.75 mL	1 mL
Atropine[a]	Conc = 0.1 mg/mL	Dose	0.02 mg/kg	0.1 mg	0.1 mg	0.1 mg	0.15 mg	0.2 mg
Administer IV/IO		Volume	0.2 mL/kg	1 mL	1 mL	1 mL	1.5 mL	2 mL
Calcium Chloride 10%	Conc = 100 mg/mL	Dose	20 mg/kg	40 mg	60 mg	100 mg	150 mg	200 mg
Administer IV/IO very slowly (1 mL/min)		Volume	0.2 mL/kg	0.4 mL	0.6 mL	1 mL	1.5 mL	2 mL
Dextrose 10%	Conc = 0.1 g/mL	Dose	0.5 g/kg	1 g	1.5 g	2.5 g	3.8 g	5 g
Administer IV/IO over 1 minute		Volume	5 mL/kg	10 mL	15 mL	25 mL	38 mL	50 mL
[IV] EPINEPHrine (Syringe) Administer IV/IO	Conc = 0.1 mg/mL	Dose	0.01 mg/kg	0.02 mg	0.03 mg	0.05 mg	0.075 mg	0.1 mg
		Volume	0.1 mL/kg	0.2 mL	0.3 mL	0.5 mL	0.75 mL	1 mL
[ET tube] EPINEPHrine (Vial) Administer per ETT only	Conc = 1 mg/mL	Dose	0.1 mg/kg	0.2 mg	0.3 mg	0.5 mg	0.75 mg	1 mg
		Volume	0.1 mL/kg	0.2 mL	0.3 mL	0.5 mL	0.75 mL	1 mL
[IM] EPINEPHrine IM preferred (Vial) Administer IM/SQ FOR ANAPHYLAXIS	Conc = 1 mg/mL	Dose	Standardized dose for Anaphylaxis	0.1 mg	0.1 mg	0.1 mg	0.1 mg	0.1 mg
		Volume	Standardized dose for Anaphylaxis	0.1 mL	0.1 mL	0.1 mL	0.1 mL	0.1 mL
Lidocaine	Conc = 20 mg/mL	Dose	1 mg/kg	2 mg	3 mg	5 mg	8 mg	10 mg
Administer IV/IO		Volume	0.05 mL/kg	0.1 mL	0.15 mL	0.25 mL	0.4 mL	0.5 mL
Magnesium Sulfate Dilute with 0.9% NaCl	Conc = 500 mg/mL	Dose	25 mg/kg	50 mg	75 mg	125 mg	200 mg	250 mg
Administer IV/IO		Volume	0.05 mL/kg	0.1 mL	0.15 mL	0.25 mL	0.4 mL	0.5 mL
		Dilute with 0.9% NaCl			Dilute in 0.9% NaCl 10 mL			
Naloxone (total reversal)	Conc = 0.4 mg/mL	Dose	0.1 mg/kg	0.2 mg	0.3 mg	0.5 mg	0.76 mg	1 mg
Administer IV/IO/ETT		Volume	0.25 mL/kg	0.5 mL	0.75 mL	1.25 mL	1.9 mL	2.5 mL
Naloxone (partial reversal)	Conc = 0.4 mg/mL	Dose	0.01 mg/kg	0.02 mg	0.04 mg	0.06 mg	0.08 mg	0.1 mg
Administer IV/IO/ETT		Volume	0.025 mL/kg	0.05 mL	0.1 mL	0.15 mL	0.2 mL	0.25 mL
Sodium Bicarbonate 8.4% Dilute with 0.9% NaCl	Conc = 1 mEq/mL	Dose	1 mEq/kg	2 mEq	3 mEq	5 mEq	7.5 mEq	10 mEq
Administer IV/IO		Volume	1 mL/kg	2 mL	3 mL	5 mL	7.5 mL	10 mL
		Dilute w/ 0.9% NaCl	1 mL/kg	2 mL	3 mL	5 mL	7.5 mL	10 mL

Initiated by / Date: _____

Rechecked by / Date: _____

Fig. 1. Single drug reference sheet with multiple patient weights. [a]Atropine and vasopressin may be administered via ETT at 2 - 2.5 times IV/IO dose. Defibrillate 2 joules/kg Cardioversion 0.5 joules/kg. [b]Round to the nearest standardized weight: round down for patient weights less than half way between standardized weight, and round up for patient weights greater than or equal to half way between standardized weights.

use simulation-based training programs in all settings wherein pediatric patients receive care.

Extracorporeal cardiopulmonary resuscitation. Extracorporeal CPR (ECPR) refers to the rapid deployment of extracorporeal membrane oxygenation (ECMO) to support tissue perfusion when conventional CPR is not effective in achieving ROSC.[17] In pediatrics, ECPR is used most frequently after postoperative IHCA associated with congenital heart disease and low cardiac output or arrhythmias.[18] Current AHA recommendations state that ECPR may be considered for pediatric patients with cardiac diagnoses who have IHCA in settings with existing ECMO protocols, expertise, and equipment.[8] There is insufficient evidence to suggest for or against the use of ECPR for pediatric patients experiencing out-of-hospital cardiac arrest or pediatric patients with noncardiac disease experiencing IHCA refractory to conventional CPR.[8]

Cessation of resuscitation. The decision to terminate the team's resuscitation effort for a child is often complicated and challenging. Many factors are considered in the decision to terminate resuscitation. These may include medical factors, such as the duration of the arrest, resuscitation mechanics, cause of the arrest, patients' prognosis, or nonmedical considerations such as parent-related factors or providers' beliefs.[19] In children, there are no concrete guidelines on when to terminate resuscitative efforts, which may lead to increased uncertainty and distress for providers involved in the resuscitation.

Family presence

Current research supports the option for families to be present at the bedside during pediatric resuscitation.[13,20–22] The American Academy of Pediatrics, American College of Emergency Physicians, American Association of Critical Care Nurses, and

Emergency Resuscitation Drugs

	Concentration	Standard Dose	Dose to be Given	Volume to Draw Up	Administer
			10 kg		
Adenosine	3 mg/mL	0.1 mg/kg	1 mg *May double for 2nd dose	0.3 mL	Rapid IVP
Amiodarone - *pulseless arrest*	50 mg/mL	5 mg/kg	50 mg	1 mL Dilute in 10-20 mL D5W	IVP
Amiodarone - *perfusing rhythm*	50 mg/mL	5 mg/kg	50 mg	1 mL Dilute in 20 mL D5W	IV Over 20-60 min
Atropine*	0.1 mg/mL	0.02 mg/kg	0.2 mg	2 mL	Rapid IVP
Calcium Chloride 10%	100 mg/mL	20 mg/kg	200 mg	2 mL	IV over 5 min Arrest slow IVP
Dextrose 50%	0.5 grams/mL	0.5 grams/kg	5 grams	10 mL PIV: Dilute with 10 mL NS	IVP Slowly
EPINEPHrine* Standard IV Dose NOTE CONCENTRATION *(see below for IM Anaphylaxis dosing)*	0.1 mg/mL	0.01 mg/kg Q 3-5 minutes	0.1 mg	1 mL	IVP
Intralipid 20% *(for local anesthetic toxicity) Stored in Omnicell*	200 mg/mL	1.5 mL/kg	15 mL	15 mL	IV over 1 min May repeat x1 after 5 min
Lidocaine*	20 mg/mL	1 mg/kg	10 mg	0.5 mL	IVP
Magnesium Sulfate	500 mg/mL	50 mg/kg	500 mg	1 mL Dilute in 10 mL NS	IV over 20min Arrest: IVP
Sodium Bicarbonate	1 mEq/mL	1 mEq/kg	10 mEq	10 mL	IVP Slowly
Anaphylaxis					
EPINEPHrine Anaphylaxis IM NOTE CONCENTRATION *(see above for standard IV dosing)*	1 mg/mL	0.01 mg/kg Q5-15 minutes	0.1 mg	0.1 mL	Intramuscular (IM) - Anaphylaxis Dosing Only
Reversal Agents - Doses listed are for full reversal					
Naloxone (Narcan)*	0.4 mg/mL	0.1 mg/kg	1 mg	2.5 mL	IVP over 30 sec
Flumazenil (Romazicon)	0.1 mg/mL	0.01 mg/kg	0.1 mg	1 mL	IVP over 30 sec
Anticonvulsant - Status Epilepticus					
Lorazepam (Ativan) - in Omnicell	2 mg/mL	0.1 mg/kg	1 mg	0.5 mL Dilute to 1mg/mL (NS, D5W or SWFI)	2-5 min IVP
Intubating Agents					
Fentanyl - in Omnicell	50 mcg/mL	1 to 3 mcg/kg	10 to 30 mcg	0.2 mL to 0.6 mL	3-5 min IVP
Midazolam (Versed) - in omnicell	1 mg/mL	0.05 to 0.1 mg/kg	0.5 to 1 mg	0.5 mL to 1 mL	2-5 min IVP
Propofol (Diprivan) - in Omnicell	10 mg/mL	0.5 to 3 mg/kg	5 to 30 mg	0.5 mL to 3 mL	20-30 sec IVP
Rocuronium - in Omnicell	10 mg/mL	1 to 1.5 mg/kg	10 to 15 mg	1 mL to 1.5 mL	Rapid IVP
*Endotracheal Administration Dosing (when indicated - IV/IO route preferred)					
Atropine* Endotracheal (ETT)	0.1 mg/mL	0.04 mg/kg	0.4 mg	4 mL	
EPINEPHrine* Endotracheal (ETT) NOTE CONCENTRATION	1 mg/mL	0.1 mg/kg	1 mg	1 mL Dilute in 1-2 mL NS	Via tracheal tube. Flush with 2 mL NS followed by 5 manual ventilations.
Lidocaine* Endotracheal (ETT)	20 mg/mL	2 mg/kg	20 mg	1 mL Dilute in 1-2 mL NS	
Naloxone (Narcan)* Endotracheal (ETT)	0.4 mg/mL	0.2 mg/kg	2 mg	5 mL Dilute in 1-2 mL NS	
Miscellaneous					
Fluid Bolus	10 to 20 mL/kg	100 mL to 200 mL		LMA Size	Size 1.5 or 2
Defibrillation	1st shock	20 joules		ETT Size	3.5
	2nd shock	40 joules		Intubation Blade Size	1
	thereafter...	40 joules		Foley Size	8-10 fr
Cardioversion	0.5-1 joules/kg; may increase to 2 j/kg			NG Tube Size	8-10 fr

Fig. 2. Specific sheet for each kilogram of body weight.

Emergency Nurses Association all currently endorse family presence during resuscitation.[23] In pediatric resuscitation, benefits of family presence may include comfort to the patient, increased parental satisfaction, increased parental sense of control, and improved coping and acceptance of death.[20,24]

When family members are present at the bedside during resuscitation, a staff member not directly involved in the resuscitation efforts must be assigned the role of a facilitator. The facilitator should remain with the family and act as a liaison between the family and the health-care team.[20] All health-care team members should be aware that the family is present, and regular updates must be provided regarding interventions and ongoing care. Any behavior that is disruptive or obstructs care may warrant removal from the clinical area.[20] Families should also have the option to leave the bedside and return as needed.[20]

POSTRESUSCITATION CARE AND MONITORING

The goals of postresuscitation care are as follows:

- Diagnose and treat the underlying cause of the arrest
- Minimize secondary injury to the heart and brain
- Support end-organ perfusion and functioning

After ROSC, the pediatric patient is at high risk of reperfusion injuries, secondary brain injuries, and ventricular arrhythmias from myocardial dysfunction and hypotension. This period requires a coordinated multidisciplinary approach wherein nurses play a crucial role, with particular attention paid to oxygenation and ventilation, hemodynamics, temperature and seizure control, and glucose and electrolyte management. **Table 3** further describes general issues of concern, goals, interventions, and monitoring parameters for pediatric patients in the postresuscitation phase of care.

Both hypoxia and hyperoxia have been associated with poor neurologic outcomes in children[25,26] because the brain does not tolerate ischemia, hyperemia, or edema, and clinicians should avoid these conditions. Inadequate or inappropriate ventilation can affect the brain. For example, hyperventilation with resultant hypocapnia can cause cerebral vasoconstriction and low perfusion, whereas hypercapnia may lead to cerebral vasodilation that contributes to increased intracranial pressure.

From a cardiovascular perspective, hypotensive shock is common after ROSC, as is myocardial stunning from increased production of inflammatory mediators and nitric oxide.[26,27] Arrhythmias, including bradycardia, can occur after ROSC. Early hypotension after successful resuscitation is associated with increased mortality.[26,28,29] Management strategies for hypotension include fluid resuscitation and inotropic and vasopressor administration, with goals of adequate blood pressure (systolic blood pressure higher than the fifth percentile for age), adequate oxygen delivery, and evidence of sufficient blood flow to the heart, brain, and other organ systems.[8,30] When possible, clinicians should monitor the patient's blood pressure continuously.

Hyperthermia is common after cardiac arrest and is associated with worse outcomes.[31] Targeted temperature management after cardiac arrest has received a great deal of attention in both pediatric and adult populations. Induced hypothermia is a strategy that maintains the patient's temperature between 32°C and 34°C. A second strategy, called controlled normothermia, has a temperature goal of 36°C to 37.5°C. The Therapeutic Hypothermia after Out of Hospital Cardiac Arrest in Children (THAPCA-OH) and Therapeutic Hypothermia after In-Hospital Cardiac Arrest in Children (THAPCA_IH) randomized controlled trials sought to determine the effect of induced hypothermia versus controlled normothermia on neurologic outcomes after pediatric cardiac arrest that occurred either in or out of the hospital.[32,33] The results from these trials found no differences in neurologic outcomes at 1 year, and therefore, the evidence does not support one temperature management strategy over the other. For children who remain comatose after cardiac arrest, current recommendations are to aggressively prevent hyperthermia (>38°C) and severe hypothermia (<32°C) while maintaining the patient at either a targeted temperature of 32 to 34°C, followed by a temperature of 36 to 37.5°C, or only a targeted temperature of 36 to 37.5°C.[8] Regardless of the temperature management strategy initiated, the nurse should continuously monitor the patient's core temperature.[8]

Table 3
Postresuscitation concerns and monitoring parameters

Area of Concern	Goals/Interventions	Monitoring Parameters
Oxygenation • Hypoxemia • Hyperoxemia	Deliver adequate oxygen (based on the underlying condition) Minimize ongoing oxidative stress	Oxygen saturation (SpO_2) Arterial blood gas (Pao_2)
Ventilation • Hyperventilation • Hypoventilation	Normal ventilation, based on the age and illness	Capnography/end-tidal CO_2 Arterial blood gas ($Paco_2$) Chest radiography
Cardiovascular support • Hypotension • Inadequate perfusion	Blood pressure >5th percentile for age Fluid resuscitation Inotropic agents[a] Vasopressors[a] Afterload reducers[a]	ECG monitoring NIRS monitoring Arterial blood pressure Central venous pressure (CVP) Central venous oxygen (SvO_2) Serum lactate Urine output Echocardiogram
Temperature management • Hyperthermia • Hypothermia	Avoid hyperthermia (>38°C) Correct hypothermia (<32°C) Consider induced hypothermia (32–34°C) or controlled normothermia (36–37.5°C), depending on the arrest etiology	Continuous core temperature monitoring (rectal, bladder, esophageal)
Neurologic support • Seizures	Prevent, identify, and treat seizures	EEG monitoring Brain imaging
Glucose/electrolyte management • Hypoglycemia • Hyperglycemia • Metabolic derangement	Normalize blood sugar and electrolytes	Blood glucose Serum lactate Serum electrolytes Creatinine Complete blood count Coagulation profile

Abbreviations: ECG, electrocardiogram; EEG, electroencephalography; NIRS, near-infrared spectroscopy.
[a] The patient's underlying cardiac function and pathology will help determine optimal drug therapy.

There is little published evidence about interventional strategies for glucose control after pediatric cardiac arrest, and both hyperglycemia and hypoglycemia can be detrimental in the postresuscitation phase of care.[34] The patient's blood sugar levels must be closely monitored, and derangements must be corrected. There are no recommendations to guide a specific serum glucose goal. Still, patients whose target is lower (80–100 mg/dL) are more likely to experience severe hypoglycemia (<40 mg/dL) than patients with a higher target of 150 to 180 mg/dL.[35] Additionally, a lower serum glucose target has not been shown to improve outcomes.[35] Metabolic derangements can occur both as a result of and as a cause of cardiac arrest and organ dysfunction. Serum electrolyte concentrations should be monitored and kept within appropriate limits.

Seizures can occur after ROSC, and they increase metabolic demand while contributing to increased intracranial pressure and secondary brain injury. Because of this, the etiology of any seizure should be evaluated and corrected, and the team should treat clinical seizures. Seizures may be subclinical and not detected unless the patient is monitored with continuous electroencephalography (cEEG).[26,36] Such monitoring should be performed as soon as possible for patients with encephalopathy after ROSC and should remain in place for 24 to 48 hours.[8] For patients undergoing hypothermia treatment, cEEG should be used until the patient has returned to normothermia for 24 hours.[37]

OUTCOMES

Outcomes for children who require CPR can vary significantly along a continuum from full recovery to severe neurologic disability to death. The chances of survival and a meaningful recovery are better for in-hospital versus out-of-hospital arrest and unwitnessed arrest.[38,39] Other factors that are associated with poor outcomes are summarized in **Box 1**. For out-of-hospital arrests, those that are witnessed with early dispatcher-assisted bystander CPR, which has an initial shockable rhythm, and ROSC within 20 minutes can potentially improve outcomes.[18]

Avoiding the need for resuscitation in the first place is one key to improving patient outcomes. Clinicians can accomplish this with early identification that the patient is decompensating while initiating interventions to prevent arrest. In the inpatient setting, tools that can help identify patient decompensation, such as the PEWS, are available.[40]

From an outpatient perspective, an increasing number of medically complex children living outside the hospital require technology such as tracheostomy tubes and home ventilation. These children are at risk of airway compromise, which can lead to cardiac arrest. Parents and caregivers in the home need specialized training to recognize distress and initiate airway management interventions, such as suctioning and changing the tube, if there is concern for obstruction or decannulation.[41] They should also be prepared to perform additional basic life support measures, such as chest compressions, while awaiting help from emergency medical services (EMSs). Local EMSs should be informed when a child with specialized medical needs lives in their community. Additional strategies for emergency response in the home include having an emergency bag available with items such as a resuscitation bag and mask, extra tracheostomy tubes and obturators, and suction catheters.[42]

Because pediatric resuscitation is a relatively rare event, team members do not have many opportunities to practice resuscitation skills in real time. As such, multidisciplinary health-care members need education and refresher training to maintain competency in basic and advanced life support skills. In addition to hands-on skills, team members should practice behavioral skills that enhance leadership and communication skills.[43] Modalities for resuscitation training include high-fidelity in situ simulation training and mock code training in the patient care environment.[44] Some devices

---

Box 1
Factors associated with poor outcomes after resuscitation

- Out-of-hospital arrest
- Unwitnessed arrest
- Longer duration of cardiopulmonary resuscitation
- Cause of arrest (eg, hypoxic injury, such as drowning)
- Pre-existing medical conditions
- Presence of a nonshockable rhythm

provide real-time CPR feedback on compression rate and depth, which can improve CPR quality. However, the effect on patient outcomes is unknown. Evaluating team performance after resuscitation events with structured debriefings can identify areas for improvement.[45,46] Improved training experiences can translate to improved patient outcomes, although more research is needed in this area.[44,47,48] Family caregivers of medically complex children also benefit from CPR training and high-fidelity simulation of tracheostomy and ventilator-related emergencies.[49]

SUMMARY

Preventing a cardiac arrest event in a child is the first and most crucial step in pediatric resuscitation. Most pediatric cardiac arrests result from respiratory failure and its resulting physiologic decompensation; therefore, nurses must be skilled at detecting and intervening when decompensation is present in children. Once an arrest occurs, adherence to the AHA PALS guidelines[7] is essential along with attention to team dynamics, supporting weight-based dosing delivery using standardized bedside reference sheets, supporting family presence, and introducing ECMO when appropriate. Once the child has survived an arrest, postresuscitation care including monitoring oxygenation and ventilation, supporting normal hemodynamics, performing temperature and seizure control, and managing glucose and electrolytes in concert with the pediatric medical team is also critical. Children who experience a cardiopulmonary arrest will have the best possible outcome if their care team is well trained and prepared and evidence-based practices are followed. There are increasing numbers of medically complex children living in community settings; therefore, the care team must train parents and caregivers in basic life support. The emergency medical services in the area should also be aware of the child's needs before an event occurs.

CLINICS CARE POINTS

- Preventing cardiac arrest is a priority
- Most children experience cardiac arrest from respiratory events
- The American Heart Association's Pediatric Advanced Life Support Guidelines are the standard of care
- Once the child has survived an arrest event, monitoring oxygenation and ventilation, supporting perfusion, monitoring blood glucose, and temperature and seizure control are the priority

DISCLOSURE

The authors have nothing to disclose.

REFERENCES

1. Tress EE, Kochanek PM, Saladino RA, et al. Cardiac arrest in children. J emergencies, Trauma Shock 2010;3(3):267–72.
2. Hayes LW, Dobyns EL, DiGiovine B, et al. A multicenter collaborative approach to reducing pediatric codes outside the ICU. Pediatrics 2012;129(3). https://doi.org/10.1542/peds.2011-0227.
3. Chapman SM, Maconochie IK. Early warning scores in paediatrics: an overview. Arch Dis Child 2019;104(4):395–9.

4. Rothman MJ, Tepas JJ, Nowalk AJ, et al. Development and validation of a continuously age-adjusted measure of patient condition for hospitalized children using the electronic medical record. J Biomed Inform 2017;66:180–93.

5. Trubey R, Huang C, Lugg-Widger FV, et al. Validity and effectiveness of paediatric early warning systems and track and trigger tools for identifying and reducing clinical deterioration in hospitalised children: a systematic review. BMJ Open 2019;9(5):1–22.

6. Dieckmann RA, Brownstein D, Gausche-Hill M. The pediatric assessment triangle: a novel approach for the rapid evaluation of children. Pediatr Emerg Care 2010;26(4):312–5.

7. American Heart Association. Pediatric advanced life support provider (PALS) manual. Dallas, TX: American Heart Association; 2020.

8. Topjian AA, Raymond TT, Atkins D, et al. Part 4: pediatric basic and advanced life support: 2020 American heart association guidelines for cardiopulmonary resuscitation and emergency cardiovascular care. Circulation 2020;142(16 2): S469–523.

9. Meaney PA, Bobrow BJ, Mancini ME, et al. Cardiopulmonary resuscitation quality: improving cardiac resuscitation outcomes both inside and outside the hospital: a consensus statement from the American heart association. Circulation 2013; 128(4):417–35.

10. Lavonas EJ, Ohshimo S, Nation K, et al. Advanced airway interventions for paediatric cardiac arrest: a systematic review and meta-analysis. Resuscitation 2019; 138(February):114–28.

11. Duff JP, Topjian AA, Berg MD, et al. 2019 American Heart Association focused update on pediatric advanced life support: an update to the American Heart Association guidelines for cardiopulmonary resuscitation and emergency cardiovascular care. Pediatrics 2020;145(1):1–15.

12. Weiss SL, Peters MJ, Alhazzani W, et al. Surviving sepsis campaign international guidelines for the management of septic shock and sepsis-associated organ dysfunction in children. Intensive Care Med 2020;46(2):10–67.

13. Remick K, Gausche-Hill M, Joseph MM, et al. Pediatric readiness in the emergency department. Pediatrics 2018;142(5). https://doi.org/10.1542/peds.2018-2459.

14. Sinha M, Lezine MW, Frechette A, et al. Weighing the pediatric patient during trauma resuscitation and its concordance with estimated weight using broselow luten emergency tape. Pediatr Emerg Care 2012;28(6):544–7.

15. Wells M, Goldstein L. Drug dosing errors in simulated paediatric emergencies – comprehensive dosing guides outperform length-based tapes with precalculated drug doses. Afr J Emerg Med 2020;10(2):74–80.

16. El-Shafy IA, Delgado J, Akerman M, et al. Closed-loop communication improves task completion in pediatric trauma resuscitation. J Surg Educ 2018;75(1):58–64.

17. Esangbedo ID, Brunetti MA, Campbell FM, et al. Pediatric extracorporeal cardiopulmonary resuscitation: a systematic Review*. *Pediatric critical care medicine*. Published online 2020;E934–43.

18. Soar J, MacOnochie I, Wyckoff MH, et al. 2019 international consensus on cardiopulmonary resuscitation and emergency cardiovascular care Science with treatment recommendations: summary from the basic life support; advanced life support; pediatric life support; Neonatal life support; education, I. Circulation 2019;140(24):E826–80.

19. Campwala RT, Schmidt AR, Chang TP, et al. Factors influencing termination of resuscitation in children: a qualitative analysis. Int J Emerg Med 2020;13(1). https://doi.org/10.1186/s12245-020-0263-6.

20. McAlvin SS, Carew-Lyons A. Family presence during resuscitation and invasive procedures in pediatric critical care: a systematic review. Am J Crit Care 2014; 23(6):477–84.

21. American Association of Critical Care Nurses. Family presence during resuscitation and invasive procedures. Crit Care Nurse 2016;36(1):e11–4.

22. Vanhoy MA, Horigan A, Stapleton SJ, et al. Clinical practice guideline: family presence. J Emerg Nurs 2019;45(1):76.e1-9.

23. Henderson DP, Knapp JF. Report of the National consensus Conference on family presence during pediatric cardiopulmonary resuscitation and procedures. J Emerg Nurs 2006;32(1):23–9.

24. Parra C, Mele M, Alonso I, et al. Parent experience in the resuscitation room: how do they feel? Eur J Pediatr 2018;177(12):1859–62.

25. del Castillo J, López-Herce J, Matamoros M, et al. Hyperoxia, hypocapnia and hypercapnia as outcome factors after cardiac arrest in children. Resuscitation 2012;83(12):1456–61.

26. Topjian AA, De Caen A, Wainwright MS, et al. Pediatric post-cardiac arrest care: a Scientific statement from the American heart association. Circulation 2019; 140(6):E194–233.

27. Jentzer JC, Chonde MD, Dezfulian C. Myocardial dysfunction and shock after cardiac arrest. Biomed Res Int 2015;2015. https://doi.org/10.1155/2015/314796.

28. Topjian AA, Telford R, Holubkov R, et al. Association of early postresuscitation hypotension with survival to discharge after targeted temperature management for pediatric out-of-hospital cardiac arrest: secondary analysis of a randomized clinical trial. JAMA Pediatr 2017;172(2):143–53.

29. Topjian AA, French B, Sutton RM, et al. Early postresuscitation hypotension is associated with increased mortality following pediatric cardiac arrest. Crit Care Med 2014;42(6):1518–23.

30. De Caen AR, Berg MD, Chameides L, et al. Part 12: pediatric advanced life support: 2015 American Heart Association guidelines update for cardiopulmonary resuscitation and emergency cardiovascular care. Circulation 2015;132(18): S526–42.

31. Bembea MM, Nadkarni VM, Diener-West M, et al. Temperature patterns in the early postresuscitation period after pediatric inhospital cardiac arrest. Pediatr Crit Care Med 2010;11(6):723–30.

32. Moler FW, Silverstein. Therapeutic hypothermia after out-of-hospital cardiac arrest in children. N Engl J Med 2015;372(20):1898–908.

33. Moler FW, Silverstein FS, Holubkov R, et al. Therapeutic hypothermia after inhospital cardiac arrest in children. N Engl J Med 2017;376(4):318–29.

34. Wintergerst KA, Buckingham B, Gandrud L, et al. Association of hypoglycemia, hyperglycemia, and glucose variability with morbidity and death in the pediatric intensive care unit. Pediatrics 2006;118(1):173–9.

35. Agus MSD, Wypij D, Hirshberg EL, et al. Tight Glycemic control in critically ill children. N Engl J Med 2017;376(8):729–41.

36. Abend NS, Gutierrez-Colina AM, Topjian AA, et al. Nonconvulsive seizures are common in critically ill children. Neurology 2011;76(12):1071–7.

37. Herman ST, Abend NS, Bleck TP, et al. Consensus statement on continuous EEG in critically Ill adults and children, part I: Indications. J Clin Neurophysiol 2015; 32(2):87–95.

38. Matos RI, Watson RS, Nadkarni VM, et al. Duration of cardiopulmonary resuscitation and illness category impact survival and neurologic outcomes for in-hospital pediatric cardiac arrests. Circulation 2013;127(4):442–51.

39. Phillips RS, Scott B, Carter SJ, et al. Systematic review and meta-analysis of outcomes after cardiopulmonary arrest in childhood. PLoS ONE 2015;10(6):1–13.

40. Akre M, Finkelstein M, Erickson M, et al. Sensitivity of the pediatric early warning score to identify patient deterioration. Pediatrics 2010;125(4). https://doi.org/10.1542/peds.2009-0338.

41. Watters KF. Tracheostomy in infants and children. Respir Care 2017;62(6):799–825.

42. Estrem B, Wall J, Paitich L, et al. The ventilator- dependent child. Home Healthc now 2020;38(2):66–74.

43. Buyck M, Manzano S, Haddad K, et al. Effects of blindfold on leadership in pediatric resuscitation simulation: a randomized trial. Front Pediatr 2019;7(FEB):1–6.

44. Armenia S, Thangamathesvaran L, Caine A, et al. The role of high-fidelity team-based simulation in acute care settings: a systematic review. Surg J 2018;04(03):e136–51.

45. Reeder RW, Girling A, Wolfe H, et al. Improving outcomes after pediatric cardiac arrest - the ICU-Resuscitation Project: study protocol for a randomized controlled trial. Trials 2018;19(1):1–10.

46. Wolfe HA, Wenger J, Sutton R, et al. Cold debriefings after in-hospital cardiac arrest in an international pediatric resuscitation quality improvement collaborative. Pediatr Qual Saf 2020;5(4):e319.

47. Andreatta P, Saxton E, Thompson M, et al. Simulation-based mock codes significantly correlate with improved pediatric patient cardiopulmonary arrest survival rates. Pediatr Crit Care Med 2011;12(1):33–8.

48. Wayne DB, Didwania A, Feinglass J, et al. Simulation-based education improves quality of care during cardiac arrest team responses at an academic teaching hospital: a case-control study. Chest 2008;133(1):56–61.

49. Thrasher J, Baker J, Ventre KM, et al. Hospital to home: a quality improvement initiative to Implement high-fidelity simulation training for caregivers of children requiring Long-term mechanical ventilation. J Pediatr Nurs 2018;38(2018):114–21.

Targeted Temperature Management After Cardiac Arrest

Nicole Kupchik, MN, RN, CCNS, CCRN-K, PCCN-K*

KEYWORDS

- Targeted temperature management • TTM • Hypothermia
- Therapeutic hypothermia • Cardiac arrest • Comatose • Neurologic impairment

KEY POINTS

- Neurologic injury is one of the main causes of mortality after cardiac arrest.
- Targeted temperature management (TTM) can provide neuroprotection after cardiac arrest.
- There are numerous side effects of TTM that nurses should be aware of and anticipate when caring for these patients.
- TTM protocols can guide bedside providers in the provision of complex care through a bundled approach.

CASE

A 54-year-old woman unexpectedly collapsed while out to dinner with her family. She received bystander cardiopulmonary resuscitation (CPR) from her husband and son. When emergency medical services (EMS) arrived, they continued high-performance CPR and identified the patient was in ventricular fibrillation. They immediately performed an unsynchronized defibrillation with 200 J. Another 2 minutes of CPR was performed, and the patient achieved return of spontaneous circulation (ROSC). An advanced airway was placed, and she was promptly transported to a local hospital with percutaneous coronary intervention capabilities.

In transit, her vital signs revealed the following:

Heart rate (HR), 88 beats/min; normal sinus rhythm
Blood pressure (BP), 92/46 (59) mm Hg
End-tidal CO_2 (EtCO$_2$), 28 mm Hg and trended up to 38 mm Hg
SpO$_2$, 96% on 40% fraction of inspired oxygen (FiO$_2$)

On arrival to the emergency department, a noncontrast head computed tomography scan was performed, which did not reveal an intracranial hemorrhage as a

Nicole Kupchik Consulting, Inc., Evergreen Health, Seattle, WA, USA
* P.O. Box 28053, Seattle, WA 98115.
E-mail address: info@kupchikconsulting.com

Crit Care Nurs Clin N Am 33 (2021) 303–317
https://doi.org/10.1016/j.cnc.2021.05.006
0899-5885/21/© 2021 Elsevier Inc. All rights reserved.

ccnursing.theclinics.com

possible cause of her arrest. A 12-lead electrocardiogram (ECG) was performed and was normal without ST segment elevation.

Laboratory tests were drawn and revealed the following results:

Lactate, 3.2 mmol/L; troponin, 0.2 ng/mL; complete blood count (CBC), normal
Glucose, 176 mg/dL; potassium, 3.9 mEq/L; magnesium, 1.9 mg/dL
Arterial blood gas (ABG): pH, 7.32; $PaCO_2$, 42 mm Hg; PaO_2, 96 mm Hg; HCO_3, 20 mEq/L

A norepinephrine (Levophed) infusion was initiated in the emergency department because her BP decreased to 88/40 mm Hg (56). The dose was increased to 20 μg/min to maintain her mean arterial pressure (MAP) greater than 65 mm Hg.

Because she was not awakening and following commands, a decision was made to implement the targeted temperature management (TTM) protocol with a target temperature of 33°C (91.4°F).

INTRODUCTION

Neurologically intact survival from out-of-hospital cardiac arrest (OHCA) depends on several factors outlined in the American Heart Association Chain of Survival. These factors include (1) rapid activation of EMS; (2) immediate bystander CPR; (3) immediate defibrillation for shockable rhythms; (4) advanced EMS care, including airway management and medications; (5) postarrest care, including hemodynamic stabilization, 12-lead ECG assessment, oxygen titration, and TTM therapy if the patient is not waking up and following commands.[1,2]

The postresuscitation phase includes a system of care necessary to optimize clinical outcomes. There are many clinical factors to prioritize in the immediate postarrest phase. Considerations include hemodynamic stabilization and support, oxygen and carbon dioxide targets, consideration for immediate cardiac catheterization, as well as neurologic protection with TTM. It is important to have a postarrest and TTM protocol to guide the complicated aspects of care (**Box 1**). Protocols should address different care areas, including the emergency department, cardiac catheterization laboratory, and critical care. Many facilities have protocols built into their electronic health records that can be helpful.

Box 1
The 2020 American Heart Association recommendations for postarrest Targeted Temperature Management

TTM is recommended for adults who do not follow commands after ROSC from an OHCA from any rhythm or IHCA from nonshockable rhythm (class 1, B-R recommendation), IHCA from shockable rhythm (class 1, B-NR recommendation)

Maintain a constant temperature between 32° and 36°C (class 1, B-R recommendation) for at least 24 hours (class 2a, B-NR recommendation)

It is reasonable to actively avoid fever after cardiac arrest (class 2b, C-LD recommendation)

Class 1 = strong recommendation, class 2a = moderate recommendation, class 2b = weak evidence. B-R, randomized data; B-NR, nonrandomized data; C-LD, limited data.

Data from Panchal A, Bartos J, Cabanas J et al. Part 3: Adult Basic and Advanced Life Support: 2020 American Heart Association Guidelines for Cardiopulmonary Resuscitation and Emergency Cardiovascular Care. Circulation 2020;142:S366-S468.

Cardiac Catheterization

The evidence is continuing to evolve to provide guidance on which patients should be taken immediately for cardiac catheterization. More than 50% of all patients with OHCA have significant coronary artery disease.[3] Patients showing ST segment elevation on the 12-lead ECG should go immediately to the cardiac cath lab.[1,4,5] However, the 12-lead ECG has poor sensitivity in identifying ischemia in all postarrest patients. In a recently published study, 33% of postarrest patients had an occluded coronary vessel despite the absence of ST segment elevation on the 12-lead ECG.[6]

Patients who do not show ST segment elevation on the 12-lead ECG may benefit from early cardiac catheterization and intervention in the first 1 to 2 days after arrest. Factors that should be considered are preceding events leading to the arrest, such as chest pain or shortness of breath, as well as cardiac risk factors.

The Coronary Angiography after Cardiac Arrest without ST-Segment Elevation (COACT) trial was the first randomized controlled trial (RCT) that evaluated the timing of cardiac catheterization in patients who experienced an OHCA and ROSC but did not have ST segment elevation on their initial 12-lead ECG.[7] There was not a statistically significant difference in mortality; those who had immediate cardiac catheterization had a 64.5% survival versus 67.2% survival with delayed angiography. Critics of the trial argue the study did not prioritize those with high cardiac risk and enrolled patients with cardiac arrest regardless of the suspected cause of arrest. Those likely to benefit from immediate cardiac catheterization and intervention include shockable arrests, known coronary artery disease, high risk for coronary artery disease, or prearrest cardiac symptoms.

Troponin levels are a poor predictor of the need for immediate cardiac catheterization. Often initial serum troponin levels are negative, because troponin level can take more than 3 hours to increase. To add to the complexity in identifying appropriate patients for catheter laboratory activation, patients experiencing a myocardial infarction can also present with an initial rhythm of pulseless electrical activity (PEA) arrest. The initial rhythm is not always predictive of the need for cardiac catheterization. Therefore, as practice and guideline recommendations currently stand, postarrest patients with ST segment elevation should be taken immediately for cardiac catheterization.[1]

Hemodynamic Stabilization

Hypotension should be avoided in the immediate postarrest phase to minimize end-organ injury. Shock and hypotension are associated with increased mortality and poor neurologic outcomes.[8] A recently published post hoc analysis of the TTH48 trial identified predictors of post-OHCA critical hypotension. The predictors included nonshockable rhythm, longer delay to ROSC, diabetes, and admission hypotension.[9]

The current American Heart Association (AHA) guidelines recommend maintaining the systolic BP at a minimum of 90 mm Hg and the MAP at 65 mm Hg.[1,2] Published data do not clearly identify the optimal BP target in the postarrest phase, so clinical expertise is warranted for ongoing assessment and patient response to therapy.

Oxygenation and CO_2 Targets

During the postarrest phase, it is recommended to titrate oxygen and FiO_2 to keep the SpO_2 92% to 98%.[1] In this phase, hypoxemia should be avoided to reduce the risk of end-organ ischemia. The AHA 2020 guidelines also recommend normalizing the $PaCO_2$ between 35 and 45 mm Hg based on data from an observational trial and 2 RCTs.[1,10–12]

TARGETED TEMPERATURE MANAGEMENT FOR NEUROLOGIC PROTECTION

Neurologic injury is one of the main causes of death for both in-hospital cardiac arrest (IHCA) and OHCA.[13] Neurologically intact survival from cardiac arrest depends on numerous factors. These factors include early identification and response with chest compressions, early and effective defibrillation for shockable rhythms, providing high-performance CPR, minimizing pauses during chest compressions, avoidance of over-ventilation and hyperventilation, and rapidly identifying and treating reversible causes. Even when all these things happen, patients sometimes incur neurologic damage.

Before 2002, the approach to care of comatose patients after cardiac arrest was one of wait and see. There were no specific evidence-based therapies to provide neurologic protection and minimize neurologic injury. In 2002, 2 landmark RCTs were published showing mild hypothermia after cardiac arrest from a shockable rhythm compared with no temperature control led to improved neurologic outcomes and decreased mortality.[14,15] The temperature target in the treatment groups ranged from 32°C to 34°C (89.6°F–93.2 °F) for a duration of 12 to 24 hours. Patients in the control group did not receive specified temperature control and many experienced fevers. Post–cardiac arrest temperature management has been recommended in comatose adults in national and international guidelines since 2005.[1,2,16]

WHY USE TARGETED TEMPERATURE MANAGEMENT?

Most morbidity and mortality after cardiac arrest is related to neurologic injury. It can manifest in the form of increased intracranial pressure, cerebral ischemia, reperfusion injury, and herniation. Subtle brain dysfunction can lead to disability in surviving patients after cardiac arrest.[13]

Table 1 outlines physiologic injury that may occur after a patient is resuscitated from cardiac arrest. These changes are often referred to as reperfusion injury.[17] The goal of TTM is to reduce cerebral metabolism and limit reperfusion injury. It is thought that neuronal necrosis can be seen within 5 hours of an arrest and apoptosis can continue for several days after an arrest. In animal studies, neurologic injury often extends for days. For this reason, temperature is managed for a minimum of 24 hours and continued with the goal of normothermia for an additional 24 to 48 hours once the TTM protocol has been completed.[1,18]

WHO SHOULD RECEIVE TARGETED TEMPERATURE MANAGEMENT?

Since 2005, the AHA and the International Liaison Committee on Resuscitation (ILCOR) have recommended TTM for resuscitated adult patients with OHCA as well as those with IHCA who do not wake up and follow commands.[1,2,16] These guidelines

---

Table 1
Physiologic mechanisms of injury after cardiac arrest

• Depleted stores of O_2 and glucose • Intracellular acidosis
• Intracellular calcium influx • Disruption in the blood-brain barrier
• Release of inflammatory mediators • Mitochondrial injury and dysfunction
• Formation of O_2 free radicals • Cellular apoptosis
• Release of glutamate

Data from Polderman K. & Herold I. Therapeutic Hypothermia and controlled normothermia in the intensive care unit: Practical considerations, side effects and cooling methods. Crit Care Med 2009; 37:1101 – 1120.

were upgraded by AHA to a Class 1, strong recommendation for shockable and non-shockable (PEA and asystole) rhythms as well as in-hospital arrests.

Patients enrolled in the 2002 RCTs experienced out-of-hospital, shockable rhythms. There was clear benefit for cooling in shockable rhythms; however, PEA and asystolic rhythms were not evaluated.[14,15] In 2019, the HYPERION trial compared 33°C with 37°C in patients experiencing cardiac arrest with initial nonshockable rhythms. Survival with favorable neurologic outcomes was higher in the group cooled to 33°C for 24 hours.[19]

WHICH TEMPERATURE SHOULD BE TARGETED?

The initial studies from 2002 compared 33°C with no temperature interventions and showed clear benefit from cooling. In the following years, many facilities successfully implemented what was then called therapeutic hypothermia. The question asked by many was: if 32°C to 34°C works, would a higher temperature dose or target be superior?

In 2013, the TTM trial compared 2 controlled temperature targets: 33°C to 36°C in patients remaining comatose after cardiac arrest. The results revealed 36°C was not superior to 33°C. There were no statistical differences in survival, neurologic outcomes, or adverse effects between the 2 temperature targets. Patients who were cooled to 33°C had 50% survival, and the 36°C had 52% survival ($P = .51$).[18]

It is important to understand the differences between the TTM trial and the original Bernard and colleagues and HACA trials published in 2002. The TTM trial compared 2 temperature targets (33°C and 36°C), whereas the Bernard and colleagues and HACA trials compared a target of 32°to 34°C with a control group that did not receive specific temperature management.[14,15] The results of the TTM trial may allow a more tailored approach to therapy. For example, if a patient is bleeding or has a prolonged QT interval, a target of 36°C may be more reasonable than 33°C.

There has been great debate about the optimal duration of TTM therapy. A recent RCT compared a 24-hour duration of therapy versus 48-hour duration and found no statistical difference in survival. Interestingly, there was a trend toward improved survival in the group that was cooled for 48 hours.[20] The current 2020 AHA recommendation is to target TTM for at least 24 hours, adding that it may be reasonable to avoid fever for an additional 48 hours.[1]

The question many experts ask; is mild hypothermia (32 - 34 C) treatment truly therapeutic or should the aim be focused on avoiding fever post arrest?

In 2021, the highly anticipated TTM-2 trial was published generating some interesting results. TTM-2 was an international RCT enrolling 1,850 patients resuscitated from OHCA to either receive a temperature target of 33°C or a goal of normothermia with early treatment of fever. The patients in the normothermia group had a temperature modulating device placed when their temperature reached 37.8 C.

There were no statistical differences in mortality from any cause at 6 months. As a secondary outcome, neurologic evaluations were conducted using the modified Rankin scale, which also demonstrated no statistical differences between patients.[21]

The patient population enrolled in the TTM-2 Trial were different than those enrolled in the HYPERION Trial. In the TTM-2 trial, over half of the patients arrested at home, over 90% were witnessed arrests and approximately 80% received bystander CPR. The median time from arrest to ROSC was 25 min in both groups. Most patients enrolled in TTM-2 arrested from a shockable rhythm (72% in the hypothermia arm and 75% in the normothermia arm) whereas the HYPERION trial evaluated those presenting with non-shockable rhythms.[19,21]

METHODS OF TARGETED TEMPERATURE MANAGEMENT

There are 3 main methods to manage the patient's temperature during the TTM therapy: with surface cooling, intravascular catheters, or esophageal devices. There are advantages and disadvantages to each method, as outlined in **Table 2**. Endovascular catheters compared with external cooling methods provide better control of temperature, but that has not translated to statistically significant improved survival or neurologic outcomes.[22,23] It comes down to the method that works best for each facility based on availability of providers or staff to initiate therapy.

Regardless of the device used, a temperature sensor measuring continuous core body temperature with a biofeedback loop to the cooling device should be used. This allows precise temperature control and avoids overshoot of the targeted temperature. Commonly used temperature sensors include esophageal probes, bladder catheters, and intravascular core temperature sensors. Based on the patient's core temperature, water circulating through the device is heated or cooled using sophisticated algorithms to provide more precise control throughout the duration of TTM therapy.

Ice packs and basic water blankets should be avoided to prevent overshoot of the target temperature. In a retrospective study, overcooling was common when these methods were used. Sixty-three percent of patients experienced temperatures less than 32°C for more than 1 hour, 28% experienced temperatures less than 31°C, and 13% reached temperatures less than 30°C.[24] Major concerns with overcooling less than 32°C include the increased risk of atrial and ventricular arrythmias as well as coagulopathy.[25–27]

The AHA does not recommend the routine use of cooled intravenous (IV) fluids in the prehospital setting to induce cooling.[1] An RCT conducted in Seattle, Washington, showed no survival benefit from infusing 2 L of 4°C saline to patients who achieved ROSC from shockable and nonshockable rhythms. The group that was randomized to iced saline had a higher incidence of pulmonary edema visualized on chest radiograph and a statistically significant increased incidence of rearrest. However, all were successfully resuscitated.[28]

Table 2			
Advantages and disadvantages of cooling methods			
	Intravascular Catheters	**Esophageal Device**	**Surface Devices**
Advantages	• Precise temperature control • Decreased risk of skin breakdown • Better control for obese patients • Can double as a central line	• Precise temperature control • Decreased risk of skin breakdown • Nurses can insert the catheter • Better control for obese patients	• Nurses can apply the pads • Easy application • Avoid invasive lines
Disadvantages	• Dependent on physician or advanced practice provider for insertion • Invasive central line • Thrombosis risk • Infection risk	• Insertion can be tricky	• Potential for skin injury • Challenging to precisely manage obese patients

Data from Refs.[22–24]

PATIENT UPDATE

The emergency department initiated the TTM protocol and transported the patient to the intensive care unit (ICU). The patient received IV fentanyl 50 μg, IV magnesium 2 g, and IV acetaminophen 1 g for shivering. In addition, warm packs were applied to her hands and feet. On assessment, there was no evidence of shivering palpated in the jaw line or peripherally.

Three hours later, the patient's vital signs:

HR, 44 beats/min; sinus bradycardia rhythm; corrected QT (QTc), 0.44 seconds
BP, 108/62 (77) mm Hg
Temperature, 33.6°C (92.4°F)
Respiration rate (RR), 14 breaths/min; set ventilator rate, 14 breaths/min
$EtCO_2$, 40 mm Hg
SpO_2, 98% on 40% FiO_2
Updated laboratory results:
Lactate, 2.6 mmol/L; glucose, 206 mg/dL
Potassium, 2.8 mEq/L; magnesium, 1.5 mg/dL
ABG: pH, 7.42; $PaCO_2$, 40 mm Hg; PaO_2, 189 mm Hg; HCO_3, 24 mEq/L

An insulin infusion was initiated, as well as potassium and magnesium replacement infusions. The norepinephrine infusion was discontinued because her MAP was consistently more than 65 mm Hg with adequate urine output. TTM therapy was continued maintaining a goal temperature of 33°C for 24 hours. The common side effects and clinical pearls of TTM therapy are discussed next.

MANAGING TARGETED TEMPERATURE MANAGEMENT

There are 3 phases of TTM therapy: the induction phase, the maintenance phase, and the rewarming phase. The goal of the induction phase is to initiate therapy and reduce the patient's temperature to the target as quickly as possible. It is important to monitor for shivering and electrolyte shifting, as well as to stabilize hemodynamics. During the maintenance phase, the target temperature is maintained with tight control, while continually assessing for and mitigating potential side effects such as shivering and electrolyte imbalances. The focus of the rewarming phase is to gradually bring the patient's temperature to normothermia for at least 48 hours and avoid fever. Important aspects of TTM are reviewed later.

Shivering is one of the most common side effects of TTM therapy regardless of the phase or temperature target and must be managed. Shivering is a counter-regulatory response to generate heat to increase the core body temperature. Shivering also increases the metabolic rate, increases systemic oxygen consumption, decreases cerebral oxygenation, and increases intracranial pressure.[29] The goal of TTM therapy is the opposite of all these side effects. There are some general common approaches to identify, prevent, and treat shivering.

Identification of shivering can be challenging in patients receiving TTM. **Table 3** outlines the Bedside Shivering Assessment Scale (BSAS). The BSAS is a validated tool used to assess the severity of shivering.[30] Shivering usually starts toward the core and can often be palpated along the patient's jawline and neck. It is can be difficult to discern shivering versus seizure activity or myoclonic movements. Continuous electroencephalogram (EEG) monitoring is often performed and can differentiate seizure activity versus shivering.

Choi and colleagues[31] developed a stepwise approach to managing shivering using the BSAS. For example, if the patient has absence of shivering and scores 0, skin

Table 3
The Bedside Shivering Assessment Scale

Score	Degree of Shivering:	Location of Shivering:
0	None	Shivering is absent on jawline, neck and chest muscles
1	Mild	Neck and thorax only
2	Moderate	Neck, thorax, and upper extremities
3	Severe	Trunk and upper and lower extremities

Adapted from Badjatia N, Strongilis E, Gordon E, et al. Metabolic impact of shivering during therapeutic temperature modulation: The Bedside Shivering Assessment Scale. Stroke. 2008;39:3242–3247.

counterwarming, buspirone, magnesium, and acetaminophen could be used to prevent and suppress shivering. If the patient scores 1 on the BSAS, a sedative or opioid is administered. For scores of 2 or 3, sedation is used, and a score of 3 may warrant the administration of a neuromuscular blocking medication. **Table 4** provides an example of pharmacologic and nonpharmacologic options to prevent and/or treat shivering.

In addition to shivering, several other physiologic changes occur during temperature management. The side effects observed in patients receiving TTM often depend on the temperature target. **Table 5** provides a comparison of side effects often clinically observed based on a target of 32°C to 34°C versus 36°C. Key points for monitoring and management related to the side effects associated with TTM therapy are outlined later.

MONITORING AND MANAGEMENT PEARLS
Shivering

- Avoid it if possible, treat it aggressively (see **Table 4**)
- Monitor the water temperature of the device; if the water temperature is decreasing, the patient may be microshivering and generating heat
- Skin counterwarming with heat packs or a total-body forced air blanket can be effective to prevent shivering by countering the peripheral feedback loop from the skin to the hypothalamus[32]

Electrolyte Shifting

- At lower temperatures (32°C–34°C), there is intracellular shifting of potassium, magnesium and phosphate[33]

Table 4
Pharmacologic and nonpharmacologic approaches to shivering management

	Pharmacologic	Nonpharmacologic

Less Aggressive	Buspirone PFT
	Magnesium IV
	Acetaminophen IV
	Opioids IV (fentanyl, meperidine)
	Sedation (propofol,
	    dexmedetomidine,
	    benzodiazepines)
		Skin counterwarming of hands
		    and feet
		Skin counterwarming with forced
		    air blanket

Most Aggressive	Neuromuscular blocking agents (cisatracurium, vecuronium)	—

Abbreviation: PFT, pulmonary function test.

Table 5 Side effects of targeted temperature management based on temperature target		
Physiologic Parameter	**32°–34°C**	**36°C**
Bradycardia	Yes, common	Not as much
Shivering	Yes, <34°C	Yes
Electrolyte shifts	Yes, especially potassium and magnesium	Not as much
Drug metabolism and clearance	Prolonged, especially propofol, benzodiazepines, neuromuscular blocking agents, heparin	Not as much
Cold-induced diuresis	Yes	Not as much

- Cold diuretic effect results in the loss of intravascular volume and loss of potassium in the urine
- Assess electrolytes every 6 hours or as needed and supplement as necessary during the induction and maintenance phases
- When rewarming, electrolytes shift back into the cell; do not replace electrolytes during the rewarming phase unless necessary
- Protocols should specify guidance on electrolyte replacement during all phases of TTM

Bradycardia

- Common at lower temperatures and usually well tolerated
- Do not treat unless symptomatic with a low MAP
- If symptomatic, consider atropine, a vasopressor with chronotropic effects, or increasing the target temperature
- Osborne waves may be visible on the ECG at lower temperatures (32°C–34°C)

QT Prolongation

- Cooling at lower temperatures can prolong the QTc interval
- Caution with concomitant use of medications that prolong the QTc interval (eg, fluoroquinolones, antipsychotic medications)

Hyperglycemia

- Postarrest physiologic stress can lead to insulin resistance at lower temperatures[33,34]
- Assess the blood glucose level throughout the protocol
- There is very little evidence on the best glucose target; most protocols follow general critical care practice to keep the glucose level less than 180 mg/dL[35,36]
- If using a lower temperature target, finger-stick glucose checks should be avoided because they may be inaccurate

Hyperlactemia

- Increased lactate level is common after cardiac arrest
- Usually clears within 24 to 48 hours, especially once the patient is rewarmed
- If there is a new increase during or after therapy, consider shock, a new infection, or ischemic bowel

Drug Metabolism

- Cooling at lower temperatures can alter drug metabolism and decrease clearance, making the neurologic examination challenging
- May see prolonged effects of medications, even after the rewarming phase
- Many medications are metabolized and excreted by the liver or kidneys
- Caution with propofol, benzodiazepines, or heparin at lower temperature targets because of decreased clearance
- Consult the provider or clinical pharmacist for dose alterations and adjustments if needed

Gastrointestinal Motility

- Slower gastrointestinal motility and decreased absorption at lower temperatures
- Tube feedings are usually avoided until therapy has concluded, especially if paralytic or neuromuscular blocking agents are used
- Oral/nasogastric tube medications may have altered absorption; consider this if Plavix, ticagrelor, or aspirin are used

Coagulopathy

- TTM at lower temperature targets can slightly prolong the activated partial thromboplastin time, although the bleeding risk is small
- If heparin is used, consult the provider or clinical pharmacist to consider dosing adjustment if lower temperatures are used as a target

Decreased Cardiac Output

- Myocardial stunning is common after cardiac arrest and can be identified with an echocardiogram
- Reduced left ventricular ejection fraction (<40%) can be observed, often for up to 5 to 7 days[37]
- It can be more severe with a prolonged pulseless arrest duration
- Many TTM protocols include cardiac evaluation either routinely or if the patient shows signs of cardiogenic shock
- Often, left ventricular function improves with time, but, if the patient is clinically unstable, support with a positive inotrope infusion such as dobutamine may be needed[38]
- In severe cases of shock, consider support with intra-aortic balloon counterpulsation, the percutaneous Impella device, or extracorporeal membrane oxygenation

Ventilation Management

- Shift to the left on the oxyhemoglobin dissociation curve with lower temperatures
- CO_2 production slows, target normal CO_2
- Hyperventilation can lead to cerebral ischemia
- Standard tidal volume: 6 to 8 mL/kg of predicted body weight
- Quickly wean FiO_2: hyperoxia may potentially damage postischemic neurons
- Monitor for signs of acute respiratory distress syndrome (ARDS) and manage appropriately[39]
- Almost half of patients meet ARDS criteria within 48 hours of admission[39]

PATIENT UPDATE

The patient was relatively stable during the maintenance phase of therapy. Her temperature was maintained at 33°C for 24 hours. The most recent vital signs and laboratory results are as follows:

HR, 42 beats/min; sinus bradycardia rhythm; QTc, 0.44 seconds
BP, 116/68 (84) mm Hg
Temperature: 33.1°C (91.5°F)
RR, 12 breaths/min; set ventilator rate is 12 breaths/min
$EtCO_2$, 42 mm Hg
SpO_2, 97% on 30% FiO_2
Updated laboratory results:
Lactate, 2.4 mmol/L; glucose, 154 mg/dL
Potassium, 3.8 mEq/L; magnesium, 2.1 mg/dL

She had an infusion of regular insulin running at 6 units per hour and the norepinephrine infusion was not needed through therapy. The FiO_2 and set rate on the ventilator were decreased in response to her SpO_2 and $EtCO_2$.

REWARMING PHASE

The decision was made to begin the rewarming phase of TTM. Although the ideal speed to rewarm from 32° to 34°C is unknown, most protocols rewarm slowly, which is done in a controlled manner using the cooling device to warm at a rate of 0.15° to 0.25°C per hour. Recently published studies are reinforcing findings in animal data, showing that rapid rewarming is associated with worse neurologic outcomes.[40,41] Once the patient has returned to a normal temperature, it is reasonable to continue therapy at a normothermia target to avoid fever for at least 48 hours after the rewarming phase is complete.[1,18,42,43]

During the rewarming phase, it is important to monitor the BP closely. Patients can experience vasodilatation, which can lead to hypotension. It is important to treat hypotension appropriately. The passive leg raise test with a stroke volume measurement may be ideal to identify fluid responsiveness and guide therapy.

PATIENT UPDATE

Forty-eight hours after the patient's initial arrest, her temperature has normalized. Sedation was turned off to conduct a neurologic assessment. Pupils were assessed using a pupillometer device revealing 2.5 to 2.8 mm with equal reactivity. She started initiating breaths greater than the set rate on the ventilator, but was not waking up or following commands.

A neurologist was consulted to assist with neuroprognostication 96 hours after therapy was initiated. A continuous EEG was performed and did not reveal seizure activity. A somatosensory evoked potentials (SSEP) test was also done and was negative. Six days after her arrest, the patient opened her eyes and purposely moved all extremities to command. Seven hours later she was successfully liberated from mechanical ventilation. She experienced short-term memory loss with the need for frequent reorientation. On day 9, her short-term memory loss cleared, and she was discharged to home the following day.

NEUROPROGNOSTICATION

In 2020, the AHA updated the Advanced Cardiovascular Life Support post–cardiac arrest guidelines and algorithm to include an approach on types and timing of neuroprognostication.[1] One of the major challenges with neuroprognostication is the lack of diagnostic testing to positively predict who will wake up after cardiac arrest. Various diagnostics combined in a multimodal approach can shed light on the chances of not waking up, but there is currently nothing that positively predicts whether a patient will wake up.

Options for diagnostic evaluation include MRI to detect hypoxic-ischemic injury, continuous EEG to identify the presence or absence of electrical brain activity, SSEP to assess the sensory pathway of electrical signals from the brain to the limbs, and the physical neurologic examination. Serum biomarkers of neuronal injury such as serum neuron-specific enolase may also be considered in addition to neurodiagnostics and the neuroexamination. Neurologists play a pivotal role in TTM therapy to assist with neuroprognostication.

SUCCESSFUL TARGETED TEMPERATURE MANAGEMENT PROGRAMS

Another important aspect of care is quality improvement by measuring data, including compliance with TTM protocols and formal review processes to provide feedback and improve care. There are a few options for standardized collection and reporting of cardiac arrest data, including the AHA Get with the Guidelines registry, the University of Penn Alliance for Therapeutic Hypothermia (PATH), and the Cardiac Arrest Registry to Enhance Survival (CARES) database.[44–46] Many successful facilities have a dedicated TTM committee that works collaboratively with the Code Blue committee.

Improving postresuscitation outcomes is achievable. Keys to success in postarrest care include having an established TTM protocol that spans across care areas; coordination of care across multiple disciplines; training of health care providers, including nursing, respiratory therapists and provider staff; and buy-in from leadership in EMS, emergency department, critical care, and the cardiac catheterization laboratory.

CLINICS CARE POINTS

- The avoidance of hypotension post cardiac arrest is essential.
- For patients remaining comatose, temperature should be managed at a pre-determined dose tailored to the patient. If lower temperatures are used as a target, it is important to manage side effects of the therapy.

DISCLOSURE

Speaker's bureau for Stryker Medical and Baxter Healthcare; consultant: Baxter Healthcare.

REFERENCES

1. Panchal A, Bartos J, Cabanas J, et al. Part 3: adult basic and advanced life support: 2020 american heart association guidelines for cardiopulmonary resuscitation and emergency cardiovascular care. Circulation 2020;142:S366–468.
2. Berg K, Soar J, Andersen L, et al, on behalf of the Adult Advanced Life Support Collaborators. Adult advanced life support: 2020 international consensus on cardiopulmonary resuscitation and emergency cardiovascular care science with treatment recommendations. Resuscitation 2020;142(suppl 1):S92–139.
3. Stub D, Bernard S, Duffy S, et al. Post cardiac arrest syndrome: a review of therapeutic strategies. Circulation 2011;123(13):1428–35.
4. Reddy S, Lee K. Role of Cardiac Catheterization Lab post resuscitation in patients with ST elevation myocardial infarction. Curr Cardiol Rev 2018;14(2):85–91.

5. Levine G, Bates E, Blankenship J, et al. 2015 ACC/AHA/SCAI focused update on primary percutaneous coronary intervention for patients with ST-elevation myocardial infarction: an update of the 2011 ACCF/AHA/SCAI guideline for percutaneous coronary intervention and the 2013 ACCF/AHA guideline for the management of ST-elevation myocardial infarction. Circulation 2016;133: 1135–47.

6. Kern K, Lotun K, Patel N, et al. DBINTCAR-cardiology registry. outcomes of comatose cardiac arrest survivors with and without ST-segment elevation myocardial infarction: importance of coronary angiography. J Am Coll Cardiol Cardiovasc Interv 2015;8:1031–40.

7. Lemkes J, Janssens G, van der Hoeven N, et al. Coronary angiography after cardiac arrest without ST-segment elevation. N Engl J Med 2019;380:1397–407.

8. Young M, Hollenbeck R, Pollock J, et al. Higher achieved mean arterial pressure during therapeutic hypothermia is not associated with neurologically intact survival following cardiac arrest. Resuscitation 2015;88:158–64.

9. Hastbacka J, Kirkrgaard H, Soreide E, et al. Severe or critical hypotension during post cardiac arrest care is associated with factors available on admission – a post hoc analysis of the TTH48 trial. J Crit Care 2021;61:186–90.

10. Wang H, Prince D, Drennan I, et al. Resuscitation Outcomes Consortium (ROC) Investigators. Post-resuscitation arterial oxygen and carbon dioxide and outcomes after out-of-hospital cardiac arrest. Resuscitation 2017;120:113–8.

11. Jakkula P, Reinikainen M, Hästbacka J, et al, the COMACARE study group. Targeting two different levels of both arterial carbon dioxide and arterial oxygen after cardiac arrest and resuscitation: a randomised pilot trial. Intensive Care Med 2018;44:2112–21.

12. Eastwood G, Schneider A, Suzuki S, et al. Targeted therapeutic mild hypercapnia after cardiac arrest: a phase II multi-centre randomised controlled trial (the CCC trial). Resuscitation 2016;104:83–90.

13. Witten L, Gardner R, Holmberg M, et al. Reasons for death in patients successfully resuscitated from out-of-hospital and in-hospital cardiac arrest. Resuscitation 2019;136:93–9.

14. Bernard S, Gray T, Buist M, et al. Treatment of comatose survivors of out-of-hospital cardiac arrest with induced hypothermia. N Engl J Med 2002;346: 557–63.

15. Hypothermia after Cardiac Arrest Study Group. Mild therapeutic hypothermia to improve the neurologic outcome after cardiac arrest. N Engl J Med 2002;346: 549–56.

16. Donnino M, Andersen L, Berg K, et al. Temperature management after cardiac arrest: an advisory statement by the advanced life support task force of the international liaison committee on resuscitation and the American Heart Association Emergency Cardiovascular Care Committee and the Council on Cardiopulmonary, Critical Care, Perioperative and Resuscitation. Circulation 2015;132: 2448–56.

17. Polderman K, Herold I. Therapeutic Hypothermia and controlled normothermia in the intensive care unit: Practical considerations, side effects and cooling methods. Crit Care Med 2009;37:1101–20.

18. Nielsen N, Wetterslev J, Cronberg T, et al, TTM Trial Investigators. Targeted temperature management at 33°C versus 36°C after cardiac arrest. N Engl J Med 2013;369:2197–206.

19. Lascarrou J, Merdji H, Le Gouge A, et al. Targeted temperature management for cardiac arrest with nonshockable rhythm. N Engl J Med 2019;381:2327–37.

20. Kirkegaard H, Soreide E, de Haas I, et al. Targeted temperature management for 48 vs 24 hours and neurologic outcome after out-of-hospital cardiac arrest, A randomized clinical trial. JAMA 2017;318(4):341–50.

21. Dankiewicz J, Cronberg T, Lilja G, et al. TTM2 Trial Investigators. Hypothermia versus Normothermia after Out-of-Hospital Cardiac Arrest. N Engl J Med. 2021 Jun 17;384(24):2283-94.

22. Glover G, Thomas R, Vamvakas G, et al. Intravascular versus surface cooling for targeted temperature management after out-of-hospital cardiac arrest – an analysis of the TTM Trial Data. Crit Care Med 2016;20(1):381–91.

23. Deye N, Cariou A, Girardie P, et al. Endovascular versus external targeted temperature management for patients with out-of-hospital cardiac arrest: a randomized, controlled study. Circulation 2015;132(3):182–93.

24. Merchant R, Abella B, Peberdy M, et al. Therapeutic hypothermia after cardiac arrest: unintentional overcooling is common using ice packs and conventional cooling blankets. Crit Care Med 2006;34:S490–4.

25. Danzl D, Pozos R. Accidental hypothermia. N Engl J Med 1994;331:1756–60.

26. Sessler D. Complications and treatment of mild hypothermia. Anesthesiology 2001;95:531–43.

27. Rohrer M, Natale A. Effect of hypothermia on the coagulation cascade. Crit Care Med 1992;20:1402–5.

28. Kim F, Nichol G, Maynard C, et al. Effect of prehospital induction of mild hypothermia on survival and neurological status among adults with cardiac arrest – a randomized clinical trial. JAMA 2014;311(1):45–52.

29. Oddo M, Frangos S, Maloney-Wilensky E, et al. Effect of shivering on brain tissue oxygenation during induced normothermia in patients with severe brain injury. Neurocrit Care 2010;12:10–6.

30. Badjatia N, Strongilis E, Gordon E, et al. Metabolic impact of shivering during therapeutic temperature modulation: the Bedside Shivering Assessment Scale. Stroke 2008;39:3242–7.

31. Choi H, Ko S, Presciutti M, et al. Prevention of shivering during therapeutic temperature modulation: the columbia anti-shivering protocol. Neurocrit Care 2011; 14(3):389–94.

32. Badjatia N, Strongilis E, Prescutti M, et al. Metabolic benefits of surface counter warming during therapeutic temperature modulation. Crit Care Med 2009;37: 1893–7.

33. Xie C, Basken R, Finger J, et al. Targeted temperature management: quantifying the extent of serum electrolyte and blood glucose shifts in post cardiac arrest patients. Ther Hypothermia Temp Manag 2020;10(1):76–81.

34. Borgquist O, Wise M, Nielsen N, et al. Dysglycemia, glycemic variability, and outcome after cardiac arrest and temperature management at 33C and 36C. Crit Care Med 2017;45(8):1337–43.

35. Oksanen T, Skrifvars M, Varpula T, et al. Strict versus moderate glucose control after resuscitation from ventricular fibrillation. Intensive Care Med 2007;33: 2093–100.

36. Jacobi J, Bircher N, Krinsley J, et al. Guidelines for the use of an insulin infusion for the management of hyperglycemia in critically ill patients. Crit Care Med 2012; 40:3251–76.

37. Yannopoulos D, Bartos J, Martin C, et al. Minnesota resuscitation consortium's advanced perfusion and reperfusion cardiac life support strategy for out-of-hospital refractory ventricular fibrillation. J Am Heart Assoc 2016;5(6):e003732.

38. Vasquez A, Kern K, Hilwig R, et al. Optimal dosing of dobutamine for treating post-resuscitation left ventricular dysfunction. Resuscitation 2004;61(2):199–207.

39. Johnson N, Caldwell E, Carlbom D, et al. The acute respiratory distress syndrome after out-of-hospital cardiac arrest: incidence, risk factors and outcomes. Resuscitation 2019;135:37–44.

40. Cho E, Lee S, Park E, et al. Pilot study on a rewarming rate of 0.15 degrees C/hr versus 0.25 degrees C/hr and outcomes in post cardiac arrest patients. Clin Exp Emerg Med 2019;6:25–30.

41. Hifumi T, Inoue A, Kokubu N, et al. Association between rewarming duration and neurological outcome in out-of-hospital cardiac arrest patients receiving therapeutic hypothermia. Resuscitation 2020;146:170–7.

42. Picetti E, Antonini M, Bartolini Y, et al. Delayed fever and neurological outcome after cardiac arrest: a retrospective clinical study. Neurocrit Care 2016;24: 163–71.

43. Bro-Jeppesen J, Hassager C, Wanscher M, et al. Post-hypothermia fever is associated with increased mortality after out-of-hospital cardiac arrest. Resuscitation 2013;84:1734–40.

44. Available at: www.heart.org/en/professional/quality-improvement/get-with-the-guidelines/get-with-the-guidelines-resuscitation, Accessed January 17, 2021.

45. Available at: www.med.upenn.edu/resuscitation/hypothermia/path.html, Accessed January 17, 2021.

46. Available at: www.health.gov/healthypeople/objectives-and-data/data-sources-and-methods/data-sources/cardiac-arrest-registry-enhance-survival-cares, Accessed January 17, 2021.

Resuscitation Team Roles and Responsibilities

In-Hospital Cardiopulmonary Arrest Teams

Laura A. De Vaux, MSN, RN, CNL*, Nancy Cassella, RN, BSN, CCRN-K, Kevin Sigovitch, MSN, RN, NE-BC

KEYWORDS

- Cardiopulmonary arrest • In-hospital • Resuscitation • Roles • Teams
- Quality Improvement

KEY POINTS

- Team performance benefits from defined roles and responsibilities within large and diverse in-hospital cardiopulmonary arrest (IHCA) teams.
- In-hospital cardiopulmonary arrest (IHCA) teams should have both leadership and clinical roles.
- Structured team debriefing for cardiopulmonary arrest events can improve patient outcomes.
- A quality improvement structure should exist that provides a continuous feedback loop to team members on quality metrics.

INTRODUCTION

Patients who experience in-hospital cardiopulmonary arrest (IHCA) often have poor outcomes.[1,2] Those outcomes are influenced by institutional factors, including the effectiveness of the responding team.[2,3] Two main types of response teams may exist in hospital settings: basic life support (BLS) trained staff providing initial interventions, and advanced cardiac life support (ACLS) teams. The interface between these two responses, and differences in discipline, experience, and skill mix, adds complexity to team dynamics. IHCA teams benefit from addressing these and other factors, which may lead to lack of clarity in role and responsibility identification and ultimately team performance.[2,4]

The application of clinical knowledge and skills by BLS and ACLS teams in dynamic emergency situations is beyond published algorithms and protocols.[5] Teams who are

Resuscitation, Department of Medicine, Yale New Haven Hospital, 20 York Street, New Haven, CT 06511, USA
* Corresponding author. Department of Medicine, St. Raphael's Campus, Yale New Haven Hospital, 218A Private Building, 1450 Chapel Street New Haven, CT 06511.
E-mail address: Laura.Devaux@ynhh.org

Crit Care Nurs Clin N Am 33 (2021) 319–331
https://doi.org/10.1016/j.cnc.2021.05.007
0899-5885/21/© 2021 Elsevier Inc. All rights reserved.

designated or dedicated, have clear roles and responsibilities, clear communication and leadership, and frequent opportunities to practice together using simulation, have better outcomes.[3] There is a disparity in research on IHCA in comparison with out-of-hospital cardiopulmonary arrest (OHCA). Strategies for how to teach, implement, and sustain these characteristics within complex hospital teams are needed.[6]

In this article, we focus on the importance of quality improvement processes, as well as roles and responsibilities for IHCA teams to support best practices. The PubMed database was searched for full-text, peer-reviewed articles published within the last 10 years using search terms "team dynamics" and "cardiopulmonary resuscitation." Three hundred and sixty seven results were scanned for relevance to in-hospital cardiac arrest and content. Fifty-seven articles were reviewed in-depth, and their reference lists also cross-checked for relevance. The search was expanded to capture articles on how debriefing and quality improvement strategies may improve team performance.

BACKGROUND/HISTORICAL CONTEXT
Quality Improvement

Each year more than 290,000 adult cardiac arrests occur in US hospitals, and only about 25% of those patients survive.[1] Quality improvement programs should focus on such interventions as didactic and simulation education, research, debriefing, team training, quality metric feedback loops, and data analysis. These programs require high-quality, standardized data to support evaluation and benchmarking among hospitals. Standard methods for collecting resuscitation data in national registries were developed to document the epidemiology of IHCA and performance on key metrics. Over time, IHCA teams have evolved in response to the feedback loop provided by these national registries, and the research they have produced.[7,8] In addition, regulatory agencies such as the Joint Commission, the American Heart Association (AHA), and the International Liaison Committee on Resuscitation (ILCOR), have held health care institutions and teams accountable by developing and monitoring for compliance with readiness to provide resuscitation, and standards of care.

Before 2000, a lack of uniformity in reporting cardiac arrest outcomes, patient population, and variables existed. To address this, the 1997 ILCOR developed and published the Utstein Style guidelines for reviewing, reporting, and conducting research on in-hospital resuscitation.[9,10] On January 1, 2000, the AHA launched the National Registry of Cardiopulmonary Resuscitation (NRCPR). The NRCPR was a voluntary, standardized performance improvement database that allowed participating hospitals to track cardiac arrests in a national registry based on the Utstein Style guidelines developed by ILCOR. For the first time, the outcomes from in-hospital resuscitation were being measured by standard criteria collected and analyzed by the NRCPR from its participating hospitals.[10]

In 2010, the NRCPR was incorporated into the AHA Get-With-The-Guidelines-Resuscitation program. This quality improvement program was now enhanced with additional tools and resources that were designed to facilitate the efficient capture, analysis, and reporting of data from inpatient cardiac arrests. This program has continued to evolve since its inception. In October of 2019, ILCOR published a consensus statement that updated the Utstein Resuscitation Registry Template for in-hospital cardiac arrest. Core elements were defined as the minimum recommended standard for quality assurance/improvement purposes, elements that all registries should try to capture and report. These now include six domains (**Table 1**).

The data from these registries have been the driving force behind changes to responses and processes in in-hospital cardiac arrest events. Although resuscitation

Table 1	
Core elements of the Utstein resuscitation registry template: in-hospital CPA	
Hospital variables	The number of hospital admissions and the number of treated cardiac arrests per calendar year
Patient variables	Age and sex
Pre-event factors	Inpatient or outpatient Medical or surgical
Cardiac arrest process elements	Date/time of arrest, event location, event witnessed, resuscitation team called, monitoring in place, chest compressions, initial rhythm, AED used, defibrillatory shock delivered, and ECPR started
Postresuscitation process	Targeted temperature management, pyrexia avoidance, coronary angiography, coronary reperfusion attempted
Core outcomes	Date/time CPR stopped, reason CPR stopped, any ROSC, 0 d survival or survival to discharge Neurologic outcome at 30 d or hospital discharge Date/time of death if before hospital discharge, organ donation

Abbreviations: AED, automated external defibrillator; CPA, cardiopulmonary arrest; CPR, cardiopulmonary resuscitation; ECPR, extracorporeal membrane oxygenation cardiopulmonary resuscitation; ROSC, return of spontaneous circulation.

algorithms were published from this process, optimal resuscitation practices extend beyond these algorithms. In fact, the ACLS Working Group states that resuscitation algorithms are "simple visual teaching tools and memory aids" that "convey only a small portion of the knowledge needed to counter cardiopulmonary emergencies."[5]

In addition to resuscitation algorithms, the Chain of Survival is another tool that supports the resuscitation processes. The Chain of Survival provides a visual cue of the sequence of events that must occur in rapid succession to maximize the chances of survival from cardiac arrest.[11-13] Each link is critical and interdependent, such that the entire chain is only as strong as its weakest link.[14] Since its inception, the Chain of Survival has been revisited to emphasize the importance of early recognition and response. In 2015, the AHA differentiated between IHCAs and OHCAs by providing separate recommendations that identify different pathways specific to each setting.[15]

Resuscitation causes, processes, and outcomes are different for OHCA and IHCA.[16] In OHCA, the care of the victim depends on community engagement and response. It is critical for community members to recognize cardiac arrest, telephone emergency response, perform cardiopulmonary resuscitation (CPR), and use an automated external defibrillator (AED). Emergency medical personnel are called to the scene, continue resuscitation, and transport the patient for stabilization and definitive management. In comparison, surveillance and prevention are critical aspects of IHCA. When an arrest occurs in-hospital, a strong multidisciplinary approach includes the teams of medical professionals already caring for the patient and those who respond to provide ACLS assessment interventions, such as rapid response, medical emergency, or resuscitation teams. The composition of the rapid response, medical emergency, and/or resuscitation teams depend on the resources, structure, and volume of emergencies per institution. Readiness of the first rescuer BLS responders in hospitals mirror the community response for OHCA. Outcomes from IHCA are superior to

OHCA, which is likely attributable, in part, to reduced delays in initiation of effective resuscitation practices and availability of skilled rescuers.

Since the first AHA Guidelines for CPR and Emergency Cardiovascular Care (ECC) were published in 1966, the guidelines have been reviewed, updated, and published periodically. In 2015, the process of 5-year updates was transitioned to an online format that uses a continuous evidence evaluation process rather than periodic reviews. This allowed for significant changes in science to be reviewed in an expedited manner and then incorporated into the guidelines if deemed appropriate. The approach for the 2020 Guidelines reflects alignment with the ILCOR and associated member councils. Varying levels of evidence reviews specific to the scientific questions consider new evidence and clinical significance. Within the new guidelines, evidence to support pit crew/high-performance team models, debriefing tools, and quality improvement structures is presented.

In-hospital resuscitation team resources vary by institution, clinical setting, day, and time. Although IHCA teams are an important link in the Chain of Survival, no standards for member composition or allocation of tasks for IHCA teams currently exist. Many IHCA teams are ad hoc with concurrent responsibilities that need to be covered by other staff or suspended when they are summoned to a cardiac arrest. Although the history of cardiopulmonary resuscitation goes back hundreds of years, defining best practices for team composition and task allocation is in its infancy.

ROLES AND RESPONSIBILITIES

There are multiple IHCA team workflows, including but not limited to: inpatient noncritical care hospital settings with BLS response handing off to the ACLS team, and ACLS teams working within perioperative, emergency department, and critical care settings providing their own internal team response. IHCA teams offer destination care; and adaptations of the pitcrew model are required to capture the dynamics and interactions among BLS providers, ACLS teams, and expert consultants.

In 2013, the AHA introduced the pit crew model to describe the people and the roles associated with high-performance teams in resuscitation care.[2,17] Implementation of this model is better described in literature for OHCA rather than IHCA.[17–22] Compared with OHCA, IHCA teams are larger, and roles can be broken down and divided into discrete BLS or ACLS provider tasks.

The basic team model has a six-person structure with roles for airway, timer/recorder, compressor, AED/defibrillator, medication administration, and team leader. The resuscitation triangle roles are designated as the compressor, AED/defibrillator, and airway, with the compressor alternating with the AED/defibrillator role. Leadership roles are designated as the team leader, medication administrator, and timer/recorder. For IHCA settings, initial BLS responders may initiate the compressor, AED/defibrillator, and airway roles, and may hand off to ACLS providers. This basic model should be adapted to local workflows, resources, protocols, and settings. We offer a few adaptations to the model for IHCA in **Figs. 1–2**, and acknowledge there are multiple potential models to incorporate all possible workflows.

Initial rescuers to a cardiopulmonary arrest event have an important role in the outcome. In-hospital, most events are witnessed by nurses, who assume the first critical roles of assessing breathing and pulse, starting chest compressions, obtaining medical emergency equipment, and activating for an ACLS team response as needed.[23] Often described as the terrifying first minutes, these initial responders need to make rapid assessments and interventions, although they may not have performed chest compressions or used an AED/defibrillator since their last formal certification training.

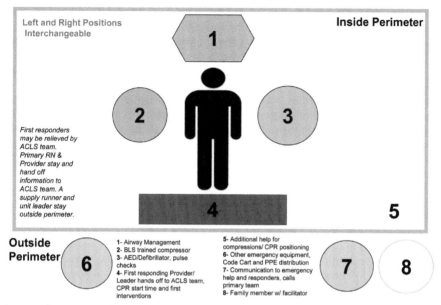

Fig. 1. In-hospital BLS/first responder roles. PPE, personal protective equipment.

In addition, the initial rescuers are likely not part of a formal response team structure, and must assume roles and responsibilities quickly in ad hoc fashion. The timing and quality of first interventions, such as chest compressions, and early defibrillation for shockable rhythms is associated with achieving return of spontaneous

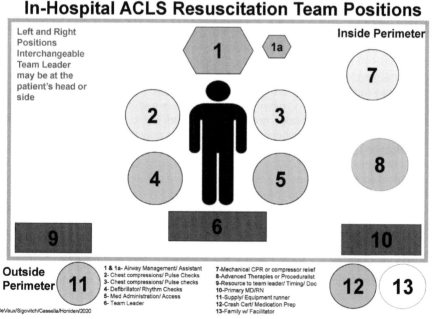

Fig. 2. In-hospital ACLS resuscitation team positions. IV, intravenous.

circulation.[14,24–26] Noting that BLS skills erode within 3 to 12 months of training, more frequent training and practice is recommended to maintain the competence to perform these skills in a medical emergency.[27] Adding leadership training to didactic and simulation education may result in better first responder performance, including the start time, rate of chest compressions, and reducing interruptions in chest compressions.[28–31]

In addition to clinical roles, nonclinical roles must also be assumed. Nonclinical tasks may include activating the ACLS team, assisting with wayfinding for the responding team, notifying the patient's primary provider or nurse if not immediately available, and supporting any family members present. Communication tasks, such as hand-off of initial interventions and patient's history, are important activities within cardiopulmonary resuscitation care, but prone to errors.[32]

ACLS team responders often arrive in staggered fashion as they pull away from primary responsibilities, assuming roles and looking for information. Summarizing information frequently can help arriving team members know what has happened so far, anticipate next steps, and identify underlying causes behind the arrest. Errors in documenting the time of collapse, whether witnessed or unwitnessed, start of compressions, and circumstances before the arrest may influence the trajectory of the resuscitation. In contrast to OHCA, much information may be known or obtained about the patient's medical history and potential underlying causes. Obtaining and conveying critical information about the patient's history from caregivers, onsite family, and the medical record to identify potential reasons behind the arrest is a key task during care. This task may be best delegated to the clinicians caring for the patient before the arrest, and/or a team resource/nurse lead role. When a BLS team hands off to the ACLS team to provide expert intervention, the primary nurse and/or provider should stay with the ACLS team for continuity of care and to prevent misinformation.

The airway role is broken down into the first BLS provider who opens the airway, applies oxygen/suction, and provides bag-mask ventilation, often performed by a respiratory care practitioner or RN. An advanced airway provider, such as anesthesiologist or intensivist, may also respond as a member of the ACLS team to intubate, or insert an airway adjunct if intubation is not desired or possible. Management of an existing endotracheal tube, tracheostomy, or laryngectomy may be required. The first airway provider can assist the advanced airway provider with equipment, suction, and bag-mask ventilation during advanced airway management. Confirmation of any artificial airway in place should be verbalized to the team. Airway providers should give feedback regarding ongoing airway assessments, as well as waveform capnography numbers to guide compression quality coaching, as well of their identification of any potential underlying causes behind the arrest which may be airway related.

Medication tasks are usually divided into preparation and administration roles, and should be performed by ACLS-trained team members familiar with the drugs available in the local emergency carts or kits, skilled in intravenous (IV) and/or intraosseous (IO) access placement and management, and practiced in closed loop communication. Medication preparation at the emergency cart can be assigned as a separate ACLS task. This role may also incorporate supply distribution from the emergency cart to the team.[34] The medication administrator should have visual and verbal contact with the team leader to receive orders using closed loop communication, and be able to provide decision support regarding medication choice and dose per algorithm providing closed loop communication for the team leader and documenter/timer. Medication preparation and timing are error prone during a resuscitation. The integration of pharmacists into the team can assist the medication roles by improving documentation and ACLS algorithm compliance.[33] Pharmacist decision support can also improve drug selection, dose, and timing activities and reduce errors.[33]

Providing compression quality feedback has emerged as an important task during resuscitation; and may be performed by the team leader or designated coach. The performance of quality chest compressions is a key factor in determining resuscitation quality and outcomes, but may often be delegated to trainees or BLS trained personnel as a physical task rather than ACLS task. Trained compressors are often abundant in the hospital setting, and incorporating back-up trained compressor resources into the team structure may reduce compressor fatigue, but may contribute to overcrowding if not managed appropriately.

Because of the potential of task overload, and number of metrics associated with measuring compression quality, identifying a designated coach can ensure this role is performed consistently. Methods of compression quality measurement may be physiologic or process, measuring the rate, depth, recoil, and minimizing interruptions in compressions.[35] These measurements are supported by audiovisual feedback devices, smartphone apps, or basic stopwatches and metronomes. Physiologic feedback including trending of waveform capnography or arterial line pressures may be incorporated.[35] The compression quality coach can coordinate the multiple data points to give clear instructions to the compressor and provide individualized feedback to optimize patient outcomes.[36]

Another role is the AED/defibrillator operator. This role may be incorporated with rhythm analysis, timing, or compression quality coaching. If the defibrillator or AED has an accelerometer, metronome, or other functionality to assist with compression quality assessment, this may fit more naturally into the defibrillator role. The AED/defibrillator role also assumes the tasks of correct application of pads or paddles, energy selection, pacing functions, and safety of delivering energy if prescribed. The operator monitors pad placement for any migration or opportunity to change placement for vectors in the case of refractory shockable rhythm. The AED/defibrillator operator should be positioned to allow for rhythm interpretation in conjunction with the team leader.

The team leader is responsible for directing care according to published algorithms, and gathering and acting on information to treat the potential underlying causes of the arrest. In addition to these critical clinical tasks, team leaders identify themselves as in charge, assign tasks to team members, summarize information frequently for arriving team members, and manage crowd control. Cooper and Wakelarn[35] found that team leaders who are able to direct care without performing hands-on tasks are able to manage the resuscitation team more efficiently.

Team leader performance may be influenced by personal characteristics, such as personality, gender, and experience; and external factors, such as the structure, training, and experience of the team members they are leading, power gradient among team members, and task overload. The team leader role is associated with a directive style of assuming control over the room and assigning roles. Inherent personality traits can influence how individuals assume the team leader role because of the perceived requirement of authoritative style.[37,38] In many institutions, trainees may assume the team leader role with experienced provider support. Power gradient between the trainee and experienced provider may result in lack of role clarity if the team and/or trainee defer to the experienced provider as the leader.[26] Resuscitation programs should explore how to address potential barriers to assuming the team leader role during training and debriefing discussions.

Team leaders may experience task overload, and some of these jobs may be delegated to other team members if those resources are available. Some institutions may have a provider and nurse leader or team leader and team leader resource role to divide up critical tasks. A transition of care often occurs when the team leader assumes responsibilities from the first clinical leader on scene. Assigning tasks appropriately also relies on a team leader who is able to identify team members and their skills. In an alternate process, team members can identify themselves, and their willingness and skills to complete specific tasks. This is done in prebriefing at the start of the shift; or may be done dynamically as the team members introduce themselves into the resuscitation.[33]

Debriefing as a tool for use before and after simulation-based education is welldescribed. Debriefing alone has been demonstrated to improve the quality of CPR in simulated cardiac arrests.[39,39] Debriefing in response to actual cardiopulmonary arrest events may take on different formats and timing. We offer two main types of debriefing in response to actual events: process debriefing and emotional debriefing. Process debriefing is used to discuss compliance with algorithms and achievement of metrics, and discuss the impact of policy, procedure, and equipment barriers to the performance of the team. Emotional debriefing is used to offer team members the opportunity to discuss difficult patient situations, including expressing feelings about participating in the high-intensity situation of resuscitation. Debriefing provides an opportunity for clinicians to learn, build teamwork, and improve performance.[40,41] Programs that offer process and emotional debriefing can support the team as a whole, and individual members. The goals of the debriefing, whether process, emotional, or both, should be outlined at the beginning of the session. A variety of members on the resuscitation team can serve as a debrief facilitator. Facilitators perform best when trained using a consistent approach; but in many organizations little training may have been provided.[42] The timing of the debrief session can present challenges, because competing priorities and other clinical responsibilities may take priority. Debriefs are arranged immediately after the event, or at a scheduled time that meets the needs of the team. The terms "hot" and "cold" debrief describe the proximity to the actual resuscitation event.[17] "Hot" debriefs occur immediately when the resuscitation event is finished. Taking a pause following an event to allow debriefing can ready team members to care for the next patient. "Cold" debriefs can occur in a more planned manner, scheduling a block of time that meets the needs of group. These kinds of debriefs could be held in a group setting or even in a feedback format that is electronic to allow anonymous information sharing.

In-hospital ACLS teams are, by design, larger and more diverse than OHCA teams. Structure, roles, and responsibilities vary depending on the size, setting, and resources available. Roles exist within these teams for the implementation of advanced therapies, such as difficult airway management, and the identification and treatment of underlying causes. In teaching, or university-based settings, the incorporation of trainees into the team structure is another nuance. Among the diversity of roles and structures for IHCA teams, the team leader role is essential in coordinating the collaborative work of these team members.

PROCESS DEBRIEFING

Process debriefing offers dedicated, interactive conversations with as many participants as possible from the interdisciplinary team. These conversations may occur individually, or in groups. Process debriefing can focus on a single event or a summary of themes from multiple events may be reviewed. Using a structured debriefing format that incorporates the key quality metrics including the time to compressions, defibrillation, first doses of medications, and the chest compression fraction can support ongoing learning and improve team performance.

Using a standard methodology including open ended questions, and citing specific examples from the events can help each team member share in the learning. A debriefing facilitator should be appointed and receive training to assume that role as part of the team. When the discussion turns to individual and team performance opportunities, the facilitator should offer suggestions in a nonpunitive and supportive manner to foster growth.[42] Process debriefs can facilitate the creation of action steps or recommendations for improvement. Structured postevent debriefing can improve CPR quality and neurologic outcomes for IHCA.[39]

EMOTIONAL DEBRIEFING

Dedicating time to express gratitude and recognition of team contributions to patient care can promote a positive atmosphere for learning. Debriefing to assist in stressors related to the event allows the team to share reactions, express emotions, and gain support from peers in a nonthreatening, confidential space. Debriefing in this manner enables groups to have discussions to normalize reactions and offers guidance to staff who may need further supports or professional services. Staff who receive the appropriate training can function as peer supporters in organizations that have a structure to facilitate their deployment or inclusion in post–cardiac arrest debriefs. Although some benefits of emotional debriefing have been demonstrated, varying opinion of the effectiveness of these peer supports exist.[39] Further research is needed to better establish the impact of emotional debriefing in practice.

RESUSCITATION QUALITY IMPROVEMENT

Development of a resuscitation quality program can support IHCA team function through data collection, performance feedback, and incorporation of the best available evidence into protocols and practice. Resuscitation quality improvement programs influence the quality of cardiac arrest care through the incorporation of epidemiologic data and population trends with consideration for team composition, policies, procedures, processes, and debriefing practices. Collecting and analyzing data on the IHCA population may expose actionable trends for the teams to address.

The people who compose the teams described previously are guided by the policies, procedures, and processes within the institutions where they practice. Problems associated with those structures can influence team dynamics and performance, and should be addressed through the resuscitation quality team or resuscitation oversight committees and leadership structures.

CLOSING

There is variety in patient outcomes following resuscitation among health care institutions. Resuscitation teams are a factor influencing those patient outcomes. IHCA teams are larger, and more complex to deliver destination care. High-functioning in-hospital teams are interdisciplinary, have designated or dedicated roles and responsibilities, and practice clinical and leadership skills routinely.[4,7] Ongoing training and regular debriefing are essential to optimizing team performance, as is the implementation of an IHCA quality improvement program to provide a feedback loop. Additional study is needed to identify best practices for the development of successful IHCA teams.

CLINICS CARE POINTS

- In-hospital resuscitation outcomes vary by institution. One factor influencing that variation is the performance of the in-hospital cardiopulmonary arrest (IHCA) team.
  - Successful IHCA teams:
    - Have access to data and quality improvement resources to provide a performance feedback loop
    - Are designated or dedicated interdisciplinary teams with defined roles and responsibilities, flexible to dynamic, time-sensitive clinical scenarios
    - Demonstrate proficiency in clinical and leadership skills, including communication
    - Participate in structured debriefing after events

ACKNOWLEDGMENTS

The authors gratefully acknowledge the following individuals for specific contributions to this work: Shyoko Honiden, MD, and Peter Kahn, MD for contributions to **Figs. 1** and **2**.

DISCLOSURE

None.

REFERENCES

1. Andersen LW, Holmberg MJ, Berg KM, et al. In-hospital cardiac arrest: a review. JAMA 2019;321(12):1200–10.
2. Meaney PA, Bobrow BJ, Mancini ME, et al, I Council on Cardiopulmonary, Critical Care, Perioperative and Resuscitation. Cardiopulmonary resuscitation quality: [Corrected] improving cardiac resuscitation outcomes both inside and outside the hospital: a consensus statement from the American Heart Association. Circulation 2013;128(4):417Y435.
3. Nallamothu BK, Guetterman TC, Harrod M, et al. Circulation. how do resuscitation teams at top-performing hospitals for in-hospital cardiac arrest succeed? A Qual Study 2018;138(2):154–63.
4. Herliz J, Bang A, Alsen B, et al. Characteristics and outcome among patients suffering from in hospital cardiac arrest in relation to the interval between collapse and start of CPR. Resuscitation 2002;53:21–7.
5. Morrison LJ, Neumar RW, Zimmerman JL, et al. Strategies for improving survival after in-hospital cardiac arrest in the United States: 2013 consensus recommendations. Circulation 2013;127:1538–63.
6. Topjian AA, Raymond TT, Atkins D, et al. Part 4: pediatric basic and advanced life support: 2020 American Heart Association Guidelines for cardiopulmonary resuscitation and emergency cardiovascular care. Circulation 2020;142(16):S469–523.
7. Kramer-Johansen J, Edelson DP, Losert H, et al. Uniform reporting of measured quality of cardiopulmonary resuscitation. Resuscitation 2007;74(3):406–17.
8. Virani SS, Alonso A, Benjamin EJ, et al. Heart disease and stroke statistics—2020 update. Circulation 2020;141(9):e139–51.
9. Cummins RO, Chamberlain D, Hazinski MF, et al. Recommended guidelines for reviewing, reporting, and conducting research on in-hospital resuscitation: the in-hospital "Utstein style". Circulation 1997;95(6):2213–39.

10. Nolan JP, Berg RA, Andersen LW, et al. Cardiac arrest and cardiopulmonary resuscitation outcome reports: update of the Utstein resuscitation registry template for in-hospital cardiac arrest: a consensus report from a task force of the International Liaison Committee on Resuscitation (American Heart Association, European Resuscitation Council, Australian and New Zealand Council on Resuscitation, Heart and Stroke Foundation of Canada, InterAmerican Heart Foundation, Resuscitation Council of Southern Africa, Resuscitation Council of Asia). Circulation 2019;140(18):e746–57.

11. Newman M. Chain of survival concept takes hold. J Emerg Med Serv 1989; 14(8):11–3.

12. Newman M. The chain of survival: converting a nation (editorial). Currents Emerg Card Care 1990;1(1):3.

13. American Heart Association in collaboration with the International Liaison Committee on Resuscitation. Part 4: the automated external defibrillator: key link in the chain of survival. In: guidelines 2000 for cardiopulmonary resuscitation and emergency cardiovascular care: international consensus on science. Circulation 2000;102(8 Suppl):I60–76.

14. Cummins RO, Ornato JP, Thies WH, et al. Improving survival from sudden cardiac arrest: the "chain of survival" concept. A statement for health professionals from the advanced cardiac life support subcommittee and the emergency cardiac care committee, American Heart Association. Circulation 1991;83(5):1832–47.

15. Ashish RP, Bartos JA, Cabanas JG, et al. IHCA chain of survival. Part 3: adult basic and advanced life support: 2020 American Heart Association Guidelines for Cardiopulmonary Resuscitation. Circulation 2020;142:S366–468.

16. Neumar RW, Shuster M, Callaway CW, et al. Part 1: executive summary: 2015 American Heart Association Guidelines update for cardiopulmonary resuscitation and emergency cardiovascular care. Circulation 2015;132(suppl 2):S315–67.

17. Spitzer CR, Evans K, Buehler J, et al. Code blue pit crew model: a novel approach to in-hospital cardiac arrest resuscitation. Resuscitation 2019;143: 158–64.

18. Colquitt JD Jr, Walker AB, Haney NS. Applying the pit crew resuscitation model to the inpatient care setting. J Nurses Prof Development 2019;35(1):E1–7.

19. Braithwaite S, Friesen JE, Hadley S, et al. A tale of three successful EMS systems. How coordinated "pit crew" procedures have helped improve cardiac arrest resuscitations in the field. JEMS 2014;(Suppl.):28–35.

20. Glendenning D. Putting the pit crew approach into practice. EMS World 2012; 41(11):41–7.

21. Hopkins CL, Burk C, Moser S, et al. Implementation of pit crew approach and cardiopulmonary resuscitation metrics for out-of-hospital cardiac arrest improves patient survival and neurological outcome. J Am Heart Assoc 2016;5(1):e002892.

22. Martin-Gill C, Guyette FX, Rittenberger JC. Effect of crew size on objective measures of resuscitation for out-of hospital cardiac arrest. Prehosp Emerg Care 2010;14(2):229–34.

23. Hunziker S, Johansson AC, Tschan F, et al. Teamwork and leadership in cardiopulmonary resuscitation. J Am Coll Cardiol 2011;57(24):2381–8.

24. Pettersen TR, Martensson AA, Jorgensen M, et al. European cardiovascular nurses and allied professionals' knowledge and practical skills regarding cardiopulmonary resuscitation. Eur J Cardiovasc Nurs 2018;17(4):336–44.

25. Fernandez Castelao E, Russo SG, Cremer S, et al. Positive impact of crisis resource management training on no-flow time and team member verbalisations

during simulated cardiopulmonary resuscitation: a randomized controlled trial. Resuscitation 2011;82(10):1338–43.

26. Ornato JP, Peberdy MA, Reid RD, et al. Impact of resuscitation system errors on survival from in-hospital cardiac arrest. Resuscitation 2012;83:63–9.

27. Greif R, Bhanji F, Bigham BL, et al. Education, implementation, and teams: 2020 international consensus on cardiopulmonary resuscitation and emergency cardiovascular care science with treatment recommendations. Circulation 2020; 142:S222–5283.

28. Hunziker S, Buhlmann C, Tschan F, et al. Brief leadership instructions improve cardiopulmonary resuscitation in a high fidelity simulation: a randomized controlled trial. Crit Care Med 2010;38(4):1086–91.

29. Abella BS, Alvarado JP, Myklebust H, et al. Quality of cardiopulmonary resuscitation during in-hospital cardiac arrest. J Am Med Assoc 2005;293(3):305–10.

30. Marsch SCU, Muller C, Marquardt K, et al. Human factors affect the quality of cardiopulmonary resuscitation in simulated cardiac arrests. Resuscitation 2003; 60:51–6.

31. Tschan F, Semmer NK, Vetterli M, et al. Developing observational categories for group process research based on task analysis: examples from research on medical emergency driven teams. In: Boos M, Kolbe M, Kappeler P, et al, editors. Coordination in human and primate groups. Berlin: Springer; 2011.

32. Bogenstaetter Y, Tschan F, Semmer NK, et al. How accurate is information transmitted to medical professionals joining a medical emergency? A simulator study. Hum Factors 2009;51:115–25.

33. Genbrugge C, Eertmans W, Salcido DD. Monitor the quality of cardiopulmonary resuscitation in 2020. Curr Opin Crit Care 2020;26(3):219–27.

34. Nassar BS, Kerber R. Improving CPR performance. CHEST 2017;152(5):1061–9.

35. Cooper S, Wakelarn A. Leadership of resuscitation teams: 'lighthouse leadership'. Resuscitation 1999;42(1):27–45.

36. Linden JA, Breaud AH, Mathews J, et al. The intersection of gender and resuscitation leadership experience in emergency medicine residents: a qualitative study. AEM Educ Train 2018;2(2):162–8.

37. Streiff S, Tschan F, Hunziker S, et al. Leadership in medical emergencies depends on gender and personality. Simulation Healthc J Soc Simulation Healthc 2011;6(2):78–83.

38. Jacobs I, Nadkarni V, Bahr J, et al. Cardiac arrest and cardiopulmonary resuscitation outcome reports: update and simplification of the Utstein templates for resuscitation registries: a statement for healthcare professionals from a task force of the International Liaison Committee on Resuscitation (American Heart Association, European Resuscitation Council, Australian Resuscitation Council, New Zealand Resuscitation Council, Heart and Stroke Foundation of Canada, InterAmerican Heart Foundation, Resuscitation Councils of Southern Africa). Circulation 2004;110:3385–97.

39. Wolfe H, Zebuhr C, Topjian AA, et al. Interdisciplinary ICU cardiac arrest debriefing improves survival outcomes. Crit Care Med 2014;42(7):1688–95.

40. Dine CJ, Gersh RE, Leary M, et al. Improving cardiopulmonary resuscitation quality and resuscitation training by combining audiovisual feedback and debriefing. Crit Care Med 2008;36(10):2817–22.

41. Yeung JHY, Ong GJ, Davies RP, et al. Factors affecting team leadership skills and their relationship with quality of cardiopulmonary resuscitation. Crit Care Med 2012;40(9):2617–21.
42. Couper K, Kimani PK, Davies RP, et al. An evaluation of three methods of in-hospital cardiac arrest educational debriefing: the cardiopulmonary resuscitation debriefing study. Resuscitation 2016;105:130–7.

Family Presence and Support During Resuscitation

Carolyn Bradley, MSN, RN, CCRN*

KEYWORDS

- Family presence • Cardiopulmonary resuscitation • Patient • Family • Support

KEY POINTS

- Family presence during cardiopulmonary resuscitation (FPDR) is a patient-centered and family-centered care intervention that is part of end-of-life care.
- The interdisciplinary team should follow evidence-based guidelines and ethical principles while offering the option of FPDR.
- FPDR is an option for the family member when the family is interested and screened as appropriate.
- FPDR should never occur without the presence of a dedicated family facilitator to support the family member.
- FPDR policies, education, and evaluation are necessary to guide practice.

INTRODUCTION

Family presence during cardiopulmonary resuscitation (FPDR) is defined as the presence of at least one family member at the patient's bedside during cardiopulmonary resuscitation (CPR).[1,2] This practice started in the acute care setting in the 1980s.[2,3] The family member is defined or designated by the patient and can be a biological relative, spouse, friend, or anyone who shares an important relationship with the patient.[2,4] Patients have the right to determine who they define as family, and who they would want to be present during resuscitation. In addition, many families feel that it is their right to be present.[1,2] There are positive benefits for families who are present, such as witnessing that everything possible was done and being able to provide comfort to their loved one, even when the patient may be unaware of their presence.[1,2] Evidence demonstrates that many patients want their family member to be present during CPR.[2] These patients often express the desire to be together with their family,[1,2,5] and to not be alone nor die alone.[5]

In addition to patients' and families' support, members of the interdisciplinary health care team are often supportive of FPDR. Despite these endorsements for FPDR, it

Heart and Vascular Center Nursing Professional Development Specialist, Yale New Haven Hospital, 20 York Street, New Haven, CT 06510, USA
* Corresponding author.
E-mail address: Carolyn.bradley@ynhh.org

Crit Care Nurs Clin N Am 33 (2021) 333–342
https://doi.org/10.1016/j.cnc.2021.05.008
0899-5885/21/© 2021 Elsevier Inc. All rights reserved.

remains a controversial practice that is inconsistently implemented in some hospital settings.[6–8] Factors that hinder FPDR include insufficient staff education,[8,9] absence of policies to guide practice,[8,9] and concerns such as perceived risks to the patient, family, and interdisciplinary team.[2,8] Such concerns are not supported by evidence. In fact, the evidence demonstrates that FPDR does not disrupt patient care, cause adverse CPR outcomes, or have a negative impact on the family member.[1,2] In fact, research demonstrates positive outcomes of FPDR for families, including reduced fear and anxiety,[1,2] fewer symptoms of posttraumatic stress disorder,[2] and facilitation of closure and grief.[1] Therefore, it is important that nurses and interdisciplinary team members are familiar with the best available evidence related to FPDR, and that evidence-based guidelines are implemented in practice. Implementation of these guidelines in practice is necessary to support optimal patient-centered and family-centered care, uphold ethical principles in practice, and optimize outcomes related to end-of-life care.

DISCUSSION
Evidence-Based Practice Guidelines

Evidence-based practice (EBP) guidelines and recommendations from national and international professional organizations such as the American Heart Association,[10] the Emergency Nursing Association,[2] the Canadian Critical Care Society,[11] the American Association of Critical-Care Nurses,[1] and the Society for Critical Care Medicine[4] support the practice of FPDR. These organizations provide evidence-based interventions for FPDR based on an extensive appraisal and synthesis of the literature. They advise that FPDR is an option for family members while taking into consideration the wishes of the patient, and that implementation of family presence follows a written hospital policy, which includes the family facilitator role.[1,2,11] Before offering FPDR to family members, they should be screened to determine if they are appropriate candidates. The team should also have a plan in place to manage and support family members who are not appropriate candidates, as well as family members whose behavior becomes disruptive and detrimental to patient care during resuscitation efforts.[10,11] There are numerous evidence-based interventions used by the family facilitator or others to support families who are present; see **Box 1**.

Interventions for Successful Practice

It is necessary to engage interdisciplinary team members who participate in CPR in discussions about why and how to implement FPDR within the hospital.[12] This can be accomplished by creating a steering committee that includes the interdisciplinary clinical staff who are involved with the care of the patient during CPR and hospital leaders who will champion and spearhead this practice change.[2,11] This committee should discusses findings from the literature, clinical practice guidelines, and professional experiences during which families were present during resuscitation. Once the committee has agreed to the task of developing an FPDR program, the group should create and implement an FPDR policy that establishes evidence-based criteria for and contraindications to FPDR (**Box 2**), roles and responsibilities including the family facilitator, a staff education plan, and a process for evaluating FPDR practice.[2,12,13] Once the program is implemented, the committee should review the evaluation data, share the data with all team members who respond to codes, and develop plans to address any areas that need improvement.

Policy

Research shows that nurses who follow an existing policy are more likely to promote the practice of FPDR.[9] However, most units do not have written FPDR policies,[1,2,9]

Box 1
Strategies for Supporting the Family Member

1. Respect the autonomy of the patient and family.

2. Respect cultural and religious decisions.

3. Stay with the family member through the entire event.

4. Screen the family member for appropriateness and interest for FPDR.

5. Advocate for the family to be within sight or touch of the patient as appropriate to the situation.

6. Maintain an awareness of the family members' reaction and meet their individual needs.

7. Explain what the family member may see, hear, or smell.

8. Anticipate comfort needs such as water, tissues, the need to sit down.

9. Recognize emotional distress and the need to walk away from the room.

10. Assist with contacting other family members.

11. Provide updates during the CPR event and communicate honestly and openly.

References: Bradley et al., 2018[12]; ENA, 2019[2]; Mureau-Haines et al., 2017[13]; Oczkowski et al., 2015[11].

---

thus failing to provide important guidance for the interdisciplinary team.[2,9] In this situation, staff must make individual decisions based on their own prior clinical experiences, values, or preferences. This results in inconsistent practice, and may contribute to moral distress.[6,7,14] Therefore, it is important that an FPDR policy is available that is accessible for staff and supported by education for all team members.

This policy should be developed by interdisciplinary members of the hospital leadership team and staff that are involved in this practice.[2,11] This may include physicians, advanced practice providers, nurses, respiratory therapists, chaplains, and social workers who respond to codes.[12] Important components of an FPDR policy include an operational definition, screening criteria, roles and responsibilities, and strategies for supporting family members (**Box 1**). An operational definition should be designed to address factors that are specific to the hospital, such as resources and staffing. **Box 3** provides a list of questions to consider when implementing FPDR. This list can be helpful in considering policy details.

Box 2
Contraindications to Family Presence During Cardiopulmonary Resuscitation (FPDR)

1. The patient does not wish to have a family member present.

2. The family member does not wish to be present.

3. The family member demonstrates a history of or current disruptive behavior, verbal outbursts, violent behavior, or is under the obvious influence of drugs or alcohol.

4. The safety of the patient, family, or team cannot be maintained.

5. There is a medical reason to restrict family presence, such as the need to open a chest at the bedside and the exposure to the sight of blood and internal organs.

6. A family facilitator is not available to stay with the family.

References: AACN, 2016[1]; Gomes et al., 2019[7]; Oczkowski et al., 2015[11]; Tennyson 2019[15].

Box 3
Factors to consider when offering FPDR

1. Is there a hospital policy to provide structure and support to this practice?

2. Is the health care team educated about FPDR?

3. Is there a prior, known patient preference about having a family member present during cardiopulmonary resuscitation (CPR) or at the end of life? If not, does the family know about the patient's wishes?

4. Is there a dedicated family facilitator available to stay with the family member?

5. Is the family member screened and appropriate for FPDR?

6. Is the family member interested in being within sight or touch of the patient during CPR?

7. Are the ethical principles upheld?

8. Is there a process in place to evaluate FPDR practice?

References: AACN, 2016[1]; ENA, 2017[2]; Lederman, 2019[22,23]; Powers, 2017[8]; Twibell et al., 2017.[24]

Family facilitator

The family facilitator is dedicated to providing family support during this crisis.[1,2,13] This role is responsible for accompanying the family member, offering the option of FPDR, and collaborating with the health care team.[13] More than 70% of staff report a greater level of comfort when there is a specific family facilitator assigned to the family member.[13] It is important to note that if the family decides not to be present, they should still be supported during this event by the family facilitator in another location, such as a waiting room.

The family facilitator role may be filled by many members of the team such as the nurse, provider, social worker, child-life specialist, spiritual care provider, or respiratory therapist.[1,11,13,15] This role can also be filled by an existing member of the code team, and does not necessarily require adding additional resources to the bedside. How the family facilitator role is operationalized is specific to the needs and available resources of an organization, and may look different between hospitals. For example, hospitals may use a current member of the code team, add a new member to fill this role, or designate a staff member from the unit to fill this role. Specific training for the family facilitator role is an essential aspect of an FPDR program and should include education related to the resuscitation process, possible family reactions, how to screen the family member for coping, and strategies to support the family members.[11,13] The family facilitator screens the family member for appropriateness before offering FPDR. The policy should clearly outline how to include or exclude a family member based on this screening process.[11] Supporting the family member is crucial, and it is essential that FPDR never occurs without the availability of a family facilitator.[7,11] The family should not be left alone at this time because it can increase distress or cause confusion and anxiety about what is occurring during the code.

Education

Another important component to an FPDR program is education of the interdisciplinary team who respond to codes.[2] Many nurses report not receiving education about FPDR,[8] which is a practice barrier. Staff who are trained, have experience, and follow a written policy are more likely to support FPDR, report self-confidence, and offer this option to family members.[8,9,11] When considering an education plan, consideration should be given to factors such as incorporating staff preferences, time, budget, and staffing.[8] Education may be delivered through online learning, interactive classroom sessions, watching videos, group discussions, case study review, role-playing, or simulation.[11,13,14] In addition, simulated code events that include FPDR improves team performance and decreases anxiety.[6] Another method is to discuss examples that include best practice such as outlined in the case study example at the end of this article.[12] To help achieve sustainability, FPDR education should be hard-wired into interdisciplinary staff orientation and ongoing competencies.[1,12]

Practice evaluation

An important component of implementing FPDR is the development of evaluation methods. This can occur through strategies such as team debriefing, peer feedback, and documentation review. Debriefing, after an actual clinical event or in the simulation setting, helps to identify concerns with individual or team performance and system issues that may affect patient safety.[16] Although the American Heart Association recommends feedback and debriefing after CPR,[17] the practice is not common.[16] In addition to providing verbal feedback, it is imperative to determine the compliance with offering FPDR and to create a plan to improve practice if FPDR is offered less than 90% of the time.[1] Documentation should include whether FPDR was offered,[1,12] if the family member decided to be present,[12,13] if there was a family facilitator present,[12,13] the location of the family during CPR,[13] the support offered to the family,[13] and, in cases in which FPDR was not offered, the reasons why FPDR was not offered.[1] A note template specific to FPDR, and available for nurses and others can help to ensure consistent documentation.[13]

Finding out why FPDR did not occur is also important.[1] These reasons may be substantiated. For example, FPDR may not have occurred because family members were screened as inappropriate, were not in the hospital at the time of CPR, declined participation, or felt they did not have the emotional capacity to witness resuscitation of their loved one. These represent appropriate reasons that FPDR did not occur. On the contrary, inappropriate reasons for not engaging in FPDR may reflect barriers and require follow-up. Examples of these reasons include lack of an available family facilitator, staff who are unaware of FPDR practice, and decisions that are made on team members' personal preferences opposed to adhering to the hospital policy. These may represent the need to address gaps in the system, infrastructure, or processes to support FPDR.

Patient-Centered and Family-Centered Care

Patient-centered and family-centered care refers to the interdisciplinary team working together with the patient and family to meet a person's holistic needs while maintaining dignity and respect, information sharing, participation, and collaboration.[18,19] There is a priority for effective communication and shared decision-making.[7] These patient-centered and family-centered care concepts are applied to FPDR when the needs and preferences of the patient and family are respected, there is a family facilitator supporting the family, and there is communication and collaboration among the interdisciplinary team, family facilitator, and family during this crisis. When providing patient-centered and family-centered care during FPDR, the interdisciplinary team must anticipate the family member's potential need to be close to the patient. The family facilitator supports families by explaining what is occurring, assisting with contacting other family members, and anticipating family members' comfort needs (see **Box 1**). During this event, a representative of the interdisciplinary team talks with the family member and is transparent about the prognosis and goals of care. The family member may have questions or additional information about the patient's wishes. During this crucial time, the interdisciplinary team must have empathy for the family who is present while they are witnessing the procedures related to resuscitation, and provide compassionate support while communicating about what is happening to the patient during CPR.[20] These key actions support patient-centered and family-centered care by connecting the patient, family, and health care team during the crisis of CPR.

Organizations that provide regulatory oversight for hospitals, such as The Joint Commission, support patient-centered and family-centered care and patient rights. This includes respecting the patient's preferences and allowing a family member to be with the patient.[21] When applied to FPDR, the hospital ensures that patient-centered and family-centered care concepts are captured in the FPDR program through staff guidance, education, and practice evaluation. Patient-centered and family-centered care should be maintained even for situations in which FPDR is not advised, such as when a safety concern or medical reason for exclusion is present. In these examples, the family facilitator needs to support the family member in another location and ensure there is adequate communication with the interdisciplinary team that is responding to the code.

ETHICAL CONCERNS

There are ethical considerations for offering FPDR. The interdisciplinary team must weigh the risks and benefits of FPDR and uphold the ethical principles of beneficence, nonmaleficence, autonomy, and justice. The principal of beneficence is supported when the team strives to do good and provides excellence in care for the patient and supportive care during FPDR for the family member.[11] This must be balanced with the principle of nonmaleficence, which is the responsibility to do no harm. Upholding the principle of nonmaleficence includes that no harm will come to the patient, who is always the first priority, and that no harm comes to the family member who is witnessing CPR. In situations that create a risk for harm, preventing harm outweighs the responsibility to do good in relation to the potential benefit of FPDR.[11] For example, an intoxicated and disruptive family member should not be allowed to be present during CPR because this behavior may disrupt patient care and cause harm to the patient. However, the health care team must avoid paternalistic decisions that exclude the family from FPDR based on personal beliefs that are not supported by the evidence.[22] Keeping the patient and family together during CPR when appropriate, respects the autonomy of the family member and the autonomy of the patient, and supports both patient and family members during a critical time that may result in death.[11,15,22] If possible, the patient's autonomy should be respected by providing the patient with the opportunity to decide if a family member should be present during CPR.[22,23]

It is important to determine the patient's preferences for FPDR when possible.[5,24] This can be determined during a code status discussion, on admission to the hospital, or in an advance directive.[5] Research shows that many patients prefer family presence.[1,5] One study exploring patient preferences on FPDR found that FPDR was important to approximately half of the participants.[5] In addition, participants felt that the patient should decide which family members could be present during CPR, and that consent should be obtained from the patient.[5]

In addition, the ethical principle of justice must be considered. Related to FPDR, justice is maintained when there is an FPDR policy and program that supports consistent practice, screening, and offering FPDR equally to all family members who are in the hospital at the time of CPR.[11] This confirms that the same option is offered to all family members, not only those who may ask if they can be present.[11] It is important to consider that families may not realize that this is an option and could miss this opportunity.

END-OF-LIFE CARE

The option for FPDR allows the family member to be present with their loved one during a critical event. The occurrence of CPR is an ominous sign related to patient survival, and the opportunity for FPDR keeps patients and families together during a life-threatening event.[11,22] Although CPR survival rates are improving, only 25.8% of adult patients who experience an in-hospital cardiac arrest survive to hospital discharge.[25] Elderly patients are even less likely to survive a CPR event.[26] While considering these outcomes, it is important to recognize that many patients do not want to die alone and prefer the presence of family.[1,2,5] In addition, most family members want to be present to comfort and support the patient, and this presence helps the family with closure and grief.[1,2,14] Research demonstrates that family members who are present during CPR experience a reduced incidence of posttraumatic stress disorder and anxiety, and would choose to be present again if given the opportunity.[1,2] Therefore, it is important that FPDR is presented as an option that keeps the patient and family together during these potential end-of-life moments.

SUMMARY

FPDR is important to patients and families who wish to stay together during the crisis of CPR. Many health care providers also support CPR; however, implementation of FPDR is inconsistent. To optimize outcomes, improvements must be made to address barriers and to implement this EBP. The priority is to provide excellent care to the patient and family during CPR, which is a potential end-of-life situation. The interdisciplinary health care team is responsible for applying ethical principles and patient-centered and family-centered care concepts to the implementation of FPDR in each situation. The creation of a policy, staff education, and practice evaluation helps to form a robust and high-performing FPDR program in the hospital setting.

CASE STUDY

Mrs Jones is a 74-year-old woman admitted to the intensive care unit (ICU) with a diagnosis of acute myocardial infarction. She is a full code and is hemodynamically unstable. Her son James is visiting at the bedside. Mary is the nurse and has worked in the ICU for the past 10 years. She is familiar with the hospital's FPDR policy. Two hours into the shift, Mrs Jones experiences a cardiac arrest while her son is at the bedside. Mary initiated emergency patient care as the code team arrived. The social worker, Thomas, served in the family facilitator role. He talked with James in the hallway. After a brief screening, Thomas determined that it was appropriate for James to be present during CPR. James was appropriately tearful, and voiced his desire to be with his mother. Thomas stayed with James during the entire event and provided care within the family facilitator role. He provided emotional support and physical comfort by explaining what James may experience within the room, being aware that he was tearful and offering a chair to sit down and a box of tissues, and helped James to call his sibling. James' presence did not impede the care of his mother provided by the team. A member of the code team updated James during the course of CPR, and explained that they were giving medications, chest compressions, and breathing support with a ventilator to help his mother's heart and breathing that were not working on their own. Ultimately, their efforts were not successful. Before stopping CPR, James was able to stand at the bedside and hold his mother's hand before the time of death was called. He was supported by the family facilitator during the entire event. James expressed that he appreciated the opportunity to be with his mother at the end of her life. They were always close and she would not have wanted to be alone.

In the electronic medical record, Mary documented that Thomas served as the family facilitator and he remained with James at the bedside throughout the resuscitation. The family location was in the patient's room, and interventions included providing James with emotional support and physical comfort, explaining what was occurring, and assisting with contacting other family members. In addition, Mary provided positive feedback to Thomas and thanked him for supporting the patient's son. During the post-code debriefing on the unit, the team discussed what went well and opportunities for improvement related to family presence. This discussion included positive feedback for the team's consistent support and attention to James' needs, and the suggestion to announce to the code team that a family member is present before coming into the room. Family presence during CPR was successfully implemented in this case study.

CLINICS CARE POINTS

- Attend training about your hospital's FPDR policy.
- Learn about and implement the family facilitator role.
- Understand how to support FPDR and patient and family centered care in a variety of situations.
- Evaluate FPDR performance and make necessary practice improvements.

DISCLOSURE

The author has nothing to disclose.

ACKNOWLEDGMENT

The author thanks Janet Parkosewich, DNSc, RN, FAHA, and Patricia Span, PhD, RNC, CPHQ, CENP, for their assistance with editorial review.

REFERENCES

1. American Association of Critical-Care Nurses [AACN]. AACN practice alert: family presence during resuscitation and invasive procedures. Crit Care Nurse 2016; 36(1):e11–4.
2. Emergency Nursing Association (ENA). 2017 Clinical Practice Guideline Committee, Vanhoy MA, Horigan A et al. Clinical practice guideline: family presence. J Emerg Nurs 2019;45(1):76.E1–29.
3. Hanson C, Strawser D. Family presence during cardiopulmonary resuscitation: Foote Hospital emergency department's nine-year perspective. J Emerg Nurs 1992;18(2):104–6.
4. Davidson JE, Aslakson RA, Long AC, et al. Guidelines for family-centered care in the neonatal, pediatric, and adult ICU. Crit Care Med 2017;45(1): 103–28.

5. Bradley C, Keithline M, Petrocelli M, et al. Perceptions of adult hospitalized patients on family presence during cardiopulmonary resuscitation. Am J Crit Care 2017;26(2):103–10.

6. Giles T, Lacey S, Muir CE. Factors influencing decision-making around family presence during resuscitation: a grounded theory study. J Adv Nurs 2016; 72(11):2706–17.

7. Gomes BD, Dowd OP, Sethares KA. Attitudes of community hospital critical care nurses toward family-witnessed resuscitation. Am J Crit Care 2019;28(2):142–8.

8. Powers KA. Educational interventions to improve support for family presence during resuscitation. Dimens Crit Care Nurs 2017;36(2):125–38.

9. Powers K, Reeve CL. Factors associated with nurses' perceptions, self-confidence, and invitations of family presence during resuscitation in the intensive care unit: a cross- sectional survey. Int J Nurs Stud 2018;87:103–12.

10. American Heart Association [AHA]. American Heart Association guidelines update for cardiopulmonary resuscitation and emergency cardiovascular care. Circulation 2015;132(suppl 2):S315–67.

11. Oczkowski SJ, Mazzetti I, Cupido C, et al, Canadian Critical Care Society. Family presence during resuscitation: A Canadian Critical Care Society position paper. Can Respir J 2015;22(4):201–5.

12. Bradley C, Parkosewich J, Chuong B. Family presence during resuscitation in the intensive care unit: strategies for implementing this policy change. Am Nurse Today 2018;13(7):17–20.

13. Mureau-Haines RM, Boes-Rossi M, Casperson SC. Family support during resuscitation: a quality improvement initiative. Crit Care Nurse 2017;37(6):14–23.

14. Toronto CE, LaRocco SA. Family perception of and experience with family presence during cardiopulmonary resuscitation: an integrative review. J Clin Nurs 2019;28(1–2):32–46.

15. Tennyson CD. Family presence during resuscitation: updated review and clinical pearls. Geriatr Nurs 2019;40(6):645–7.

16. Arriaga AF, Szyld D, Pian-Smith MCM. Real-time debriefing after critical events: exploring the gap between principle and reality. Anesthesiol Clin 2020;38(4): 801–20.

17. Cheng A, Nadkarni VM, Mancini MB, et al. Resuscitation education science: educational strategies to improve outcomes from cardiac arrest: a scientific statement from the American Heart Association. Circulation 2018;138(6):e82–122.

18. Clay AM, Parish B. Patient- and family-centered care: it's not just for pediatrics anymore. AMA J Ethics 2016;18(1):40–4.

19. Institute for Patient- and Family- Centered Care (n.d.). Patient- and family-centered care. Available at: https://www.ipfcc.org/about/pfcc.html. Accessed December 22, 2020.

20. Sak-Dankosky N, Andruszkiewicz P, Sherwood PR, et al. Preferences of patients' family regarding family-witnessed cardiopulmonary resuscitation: a qualitative perspective of intensive care patients' family members. Intensive Crit Care Nurs 2019;50:95–102.

21. The Joint Commission. The Joint Commission edition: accreditation requirements. 2021. Available at: https://e-dition.jcrinc.com/MainContent.aspx. Accessed January 11, 2021.

22. Lederman Z. Family for life and death: family presence during resuscitation. Int J Fem Approaches Bioeth 2019;12(2):149–64.

23. Lederman Z. Family presence during cardiopulmonary resuscitation. J Clin Ethics 2019;30(4):347–55.

24. Twibell R, Siela D, Riwitis C, et al. A qualitative study in nurses' and physicians' decision-making related to family presence during resuscitation. J Clin Nurs 2017;27:e320–44.
25. Virani SS, Alonso A, Benjamin EJ, et al. Heart disease and stroke statistics – 2020 update: a report from the American Heart Association. Circulation 2020;141: e139–596.
26. Hirlekar G, Karlsson T, Aune A, et al. Survival and neurological outcome in the elderly after in-hospital cardiac arrest. Resuscitation 2017;118:101–6.

Outcomes of In-hospital Cardiac Arrest
A Review of the Evidence

Justin DiLibero, DNP, APRN, CCRN-K, CCNS, ACCNS-AG, FCNS[a],*,
Kara Misto, PhD, RN[b]

KEYWORDS

- Cardiac arrest • Resuscitation • In-hospital cardiac arrest
- Advanced cardiac life support

KEY POINTS

- More than 500,000 new cases of cardiac arrest occur each year. As many as 290,000 occur in the hospital setting.
- Outcomes for in-hospital cardiac arrest (IHCA) have remained poor, with an average survival of less than 20% in 2010.
- The American Heart Association has called for an improvement in survival for IHCA to 36% by 2020.
- Critical care nurses provide care throughout the prearrest, interarrest, and postarrest periods.
- Optimizing outcomes for patients with IHCA depends on the ability to deliver the highest quality of care supported by the best available evidence.
- It is important that critical care nurses are familiar with the evidence related to IHCA.

INTRODUCTION

Each year, more than half a million people experience, and as many as 1 in 4 people die of, cardiac arrest.[1] Cardiac arrest may occur either in the hospital (in-hospital cardiac arrest [IHCA]) or in the community/out of the hospital (out-of-hospital cardiac arrest [OHCA]). IHCA accounts for up to 45% of all cases.[1] In 2017, cardiac arrest was the second leading cause of death, and IHCA alone ranked among the top 3 causes of death.[2,3]

Outcomes for IHCA have historically been poor, including a high incidence of mortality and neurologic disability. In 2010, survival from IHCA was less than 20%. At that

[a] Rhode Island College School of Nursing, Rhode Island Nurse Education Center, Office 100M, 350 Eddy Street, Providence, RI 02903, USA; [b] Rhode Island Hospital, 593 Eddy Street, Providence, RI 02903, USA
* Corresponding author.
E-mail address: jdilibero@ric.edu

Crit Care Nurs Clin N Am 33 (2021) 343–356
https://doi.org/10.1016/j.cnc.2021.05.009

time, the American Heart Association (AHA) Cardiac Arrest Care Committee called for an improvement in survival to 36% by 2020.[3] Since then, there have been multiple advances in research and practice.

As the providers with the closest proximity to the bedside, staff nurses are often the first responders to IHCA. Critical care nurses specifically play an essential role throughout the prearrest, interarrest, and postarrest periods. Therefore, it is important that critical care nurses are familiar with the evidence supporting best practices in the care of patients with IHCA. This article reviews key aspects of the literature on IHCA, including epidemiology and predictors of outcomes related to patient, systems, and treatment-related factors.

In-hospital Cardiac Arrest Versus Out-of-hospital Cardiac Arrest

For reporting purposes, OHCA refers to the loss of circulation among patients outside of the hospital, which is assessed but not necessarily treated by emergency medical services.[4] In comparison, IHCA refers to the loss of circulation with the implementation of resuscitation efforts among hospitalized patients.[5] Although as many as 290,000 cases of IHCA cases occur in the United States annually, most of the research has focused on OHCA.[5,6] In a systematic review of 92 cardiac arrest trials from 1995 to 2014, only 4% focused exclusively on IHCA.[7] Scientific advances in evidence related to OHCA are often assumed to apply to IHCA; however, important differences exist (**Table 1**). Awareness of these differences can aid clinicians in providing optimal care.

Outcomes

Important outcome measures for IHCA include survival of the initial arrest, survival to hospital discharge, and good neurologic outcome. A review of these definitions is provided here.

Table 1
Differences between out-of-hospital and in-hospital cardiac arrest

	Out of Hospital	In Hospital
Cause	Cardiac arrest is usually the primary event[8]	Cardiac arrest often results from clinical deterioration of another condition[8]
Prevention	Often impossible[5,9]	Prearrest monitoring by skilled professionals may allow the detection of clinical deterioration and implementation of early interventions to prevent cardiac arrest[5,9]
First Responders	Layperson or EMS provider[9]	Health care professionals, often nurses[9]
Timing of BLS	May be implemented immediately by layperson responder or delayed until EMS arrival[9]	Immediate[9]
Timing of ACLS	On average, initiated 20 min after the arrest[5]	Within 5–10 min[5]
Survival to Discharge (%)	10.4[10]	25.8[10]

Abbreviations: ACLS, advanced cardiovascular life support; BLS, basic life support; EMS, emergency medical services.
Data from Refs[5,8–10]

1. Initial survival is defined as the return of spontaneous circulation (ROSC) for at least 20 minutes in the absence of ongoing chest compressions.[11]
2. Survival to discharge is defined as survival to discharge from the hospital.
3. Good neurologic outcome is defined as a cerebral performance category (CPC) score of 1 to 2. The CPC is the most commonly used tool to evaluate neurologic outcomes following cardiac arrest, and ranges from a score of 1 to 5. A score of 1 indicates the absence of impairment, and a score of 5 indicates brain death.[12]

Get with the Guidelines: Resuscitation

In 1999, The AHA began collecting data on IHCA through the AHA's National Registry of Cardiopulmonary Resuscitation.[13] This registry became the basis for what is now the Get with the Guidelines: Resuscitation (GWTG-R), which was implemented in 2010.[13] The goal of GWTG-R is to facilitate the effective collection, analysis, and reporting of data, establish benchmarks for comparison across hospitals, and optimize quality improvement and evidence-based resuscitation practices. This database has supported many studies that have advanced understanding, and supported improvements in practice and outcomes.[14]

EPIDEMIOLOGY

Nearly 500,000 new cardiac arrest cases occur each year; a significant proportion occur among patients who are already hospitalized. The incidence of both IHCA and OHCA has increased substantially (**Fig. 1**).

Using data between 2003 and 2007 in the GWTG-R, Merchant and colleagues[15] determined a national IHCA rate of 209,000. This incidence is frequently cited, including its use in the AHA Heart Disease and Stroke Statistics 2018 Update.[1] However, evidence shows that the incidence is increasing.[15,16] Although Merchant and colleagues[15] found an average annual incidence of 209,000, they noted a significant temporal increase in incidence each year. More recently, Holmberg and colleagues[16] completed a similar study, using data in the GWTG-R registry between 2008 and 2017 to estimate the national incidence of IHCA. These investigators reported an annual incidence of 292,000, representing a 39.7% increase from the previous estimate, and noted a continued temporal increase in the incidence over the study period.

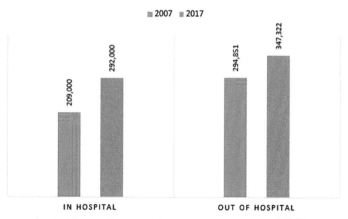

Fig. 1. Comparative incidence of IHCA and OHCA. (Data from Refs[1,15–17])

Although the incidence of both IHCA and OHCA continues to increase, outcomes differ significantly. Survival to hospital discharge for adult patients with OHCA was 10.4% in 2018 and has remained relatively unchanged over the past decade.[10] In comparison, outcomes for IHCA have continued to improve since 2000 (**Fig. 2**).

Note that, although outcomes for IHCA are improving, significant variation exists. For example, initial survival of IHCA ranges from less than 45% to greater than 85%,[18–21] survival to hospital discharge ranges from less than 10% to greater than 35%,[1,20,21] survival with good neurologic outcome ranges from 7% to 35%,[20] and 1-year survival ranges from less than 5% to greater than 35%.[20,22] Understanding the factors contributing to such variation is important to informing practice.

A myriad of factors at the patient, system, and treatment levels contribute to the wide variation in outcomes for IHCA. **Box 1** provides an overview of these factors. Some factors are modifiable, whereas others are not. Understanding both modifiable and nonmodifiable risk factors can help providers identify patients at high risk and develop appropriate strategies to optimize outcomes.

PATIENT FACTORS
Gender

Men are more likely to experience IHCA, representing 56% to 60% of cases.[24,25] Women show slightly higher rates of survival to hospital discharge, although differences in survival between men and women are minimal.[22,26]

Age

Most cases of IHCA occur among older adults, with more than 80% of IHCA occurring among patients aged 50 years or older.[23,27] Survival to hospital discharge decreases with age, showing statistically significant differences among patients aged 70 years or older, and the lowest survival rate among patients aged 80 years or older.[18] Although survival to discharge is lower among older adults, long-term outcomes among older adult survivors of IHCA are positive. Chan and colleagues[28] reported a 1-year survival of 63.7%, 58.6%, and 49.7% respectively for patients aged 65 to 74 years, 75 to 84 years, and greater than 85 years.

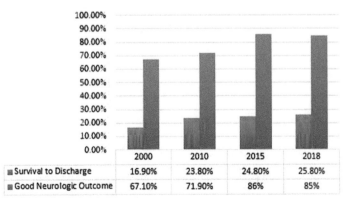

	2000	2010	2015	2018
Survival to Discharge	16.90%	23.80%	24.80%	25.80%
Good Neurologic Outcome	67.10%	71.90%	86%	85%

Fig. 2. Trends in outcomes of IHCA. (Data from American Heart Association. Heart disease and stroke statistics - 2020 update: A report from the American Heart Association. Circulation 2020;141: e139-e469. https://doi.org/10.1161/CIR.0000000000000757 and Girotra S, Nallamothu B, Spertus J, et al. Trends in survival after in-hospital cardiac arrest. The N Engl J Med 2012;367: 1912-1920.)

Box 1
Factors affecting outcomes of in-hospital cardiac arrest

Patient factors
  Age
  Gender
  Race
  Cause
  Initial rhythm
  Comorbidities

System factors
  Location of arrest
  Region
  Arrest incidence
  Time/day
  Staffing

Treatment factors
  Early recognition/prevention
  Cardiopulmonary resuscitation quality
  Early defibrillation
  Early epinephrine administration
  Targeted temperature management
  Postresuscitation care

Data from Refs[1,20,23]

Race

Racial differences in outcomes have been reported; however, this gap is closing, and more recent evidence suggests that current racial disparities in outcomes are primarily attributed to hospital-level differences in care.[1,29] In a study to evaluate temporal changes in the racial survival gap after IHCA, Lee and colleagues[29] found that black patients had a lower unadjusted survival to discharge compared with white patients (15.4% vs 19.9%, P<.001); however, findings from this study showed significant improvements over time. Specifically, the increase in survival for black patients was greater than for white patients. When adjusted for risk factors, the absolute difference in survival between black and white patients improved from 4.5% in 2000 to 1.8% in 2014.[29] The absolute difference in immediate survival improved from 2.3% in 2000 to −0.01% in 2014.[29] Study findings also showed that, although outcomes improved over time across all hospitals, the most significant improvements occurred among hospitals caring for a higher percentage of black patients. Overall, this study highlights an improvement in the quality of care for black patients and a closing racial gap.

Causes

Historically, the cause of cardiac arrest has been categorized as cardiac or noncardiac; however, causes are more varied and specific. In a study exploring arrest causes, Chen and colleagues[30] identified 14 distinct causes of cardiac arrest, including cardiac causes, respiratory causes, and causes related to other factors. Cardiac causes alone include specific conditions such as acute coronary syndrome, congenital arrhythmias, cardiomyopathy, structural heart disease, and left or right ventricular failure. Respiratory causes include upper airway obstruction and respiratory

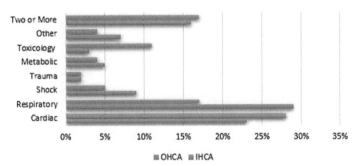

Fig. 3. Comparison of causes between IHCA and OHCA. (Data from Chen N, Callaway C, Guyette F, et al. Arrest cause among patients resuscitated from cardiac arrest. Resuscitation 2018;130: 33-40. https://doi.org/10.1016/j.resuscitation.2018.06.024)

failure.[30] **Fig. 3** presents common arrest causes and differences in incidence across causes between IHCA and OHCA.

The specific cause may be an important predictor of outcomes. Wallmuller and colleagues[31] found that patients with cardiac causes for IHCA had better outcomes than patients with noncardiac causes (44% vs 23% respectively), and Chen and colleagues[30] found a 10-fold difference in outcomes across the 14 specific causes identified in their study. There are additional considerations for certain specialty populations. For example, although the average survival to hospital discharge for IHCA is greater than 25%,[10] Fehnel and colleagues[32] reported an estimated survival of 8% among cerebrovascular patients who experienced IHCA.

In addition to differences in outcomes, consideration for the specific cause is important in guiding treatment decisions. Because certain treatments may be helpful for a given cause but ineffective or harmful for other causes, awareness of causal differences in IHCA should guide clinicians in the initial assessment and implementation of treatments tailored to the individual patient.

Underlying Rhythm

An important factor in cardiac arrest is whether the initial rhythm is shockable or nonshockable. Shockable rhythms include ventricular fibrillation (VF) and pulseless ventricular tachycardia (VT). Nonshockable rhythms include pulseless electrical activity (PEA), pseudo-PEA, and asystole.[14]

Whether the initial rhythm is shockable or nonshockable drives priorities in treatment and is an important predictor of outcomes. Approximately 15% to 20% of patients with IHCA have an initial shockable rhythm.[10,19,20] Of nonshockable rhythms, asystole accounts for more than 50%, with PEA accounting for the remainder.[10] An initial shockable rhythm is associated with improved rates of ROSC, survival to hospital discharge, and long-term outcomes **(Fig. 4)**.[19] In addition, early treatment, defined as defibrillation within 2 minutes for shockable rhythms, or administering epinephrine within 5 minutes for nonshockable rhythms, has been shown to significantly improve outcomes **(Fig. 5)**.[20,33]

Comorbidities

Several comorbidities have been shown to affect outcomes among patients with IHCA. The factors most strongly correlated with negative outcomes include sepsis, hypotension, metastatic or hematologic malignancy, and renal, hepatic, or respiratory

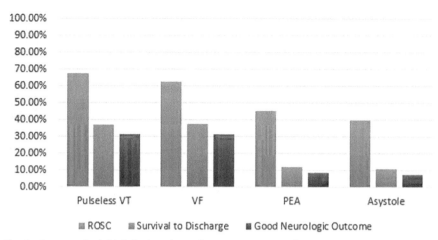

Fig. 4. Outcome by initial rhythm. (Data from Meaney P, Nadkarni V, Kern K, et al. Rhythms and outcomes of adult in-hospital cardiac arrest. Crit Care Med 2010;38: 101-108.)

insufficiency.[18,23,27] In addition, requirements for prearrest mechanical ventilation or vasopressor support are associated with the reduced achievement of ROSC and survival to discharge.[18] Conditions associated with improved survival include diabetes, acute myocardial infarction, and dysrhythmia.[22,25,26]

SYSTEM FACTORS
Arrest Location

Several system-level factors have been associated with cardiac arrest outcomes, as outlined in **Box 1**. One important system factor is whether the arrest occurs in a monitored or nonmonitored unit. IHCA occurring in an intensive care unit (ICU) or other monitored unit is associated with improved outcomes, including higher rates of ROSC, survival to hospital discharge, and good neurologic outcomes.[18,23,27,34]

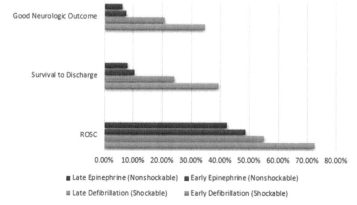

Fig. 5. Impact of early versus late defibrillation or epinephrine. (Data from Patel K, Spertus J, Khariton Y, et al. Association between prompt defibrillation and epinephrine treatment with long-term survival after in-hospital cardiac arrest. Circulation 2018;137:2041-2051. https://doi.org/10.1161/CIRCULATIONAHA.117.030488)

To evaluate differences in outcomes of IHCA based on arrest location, Perman and colleagues[34] conducted a retrospective study of 85,201 IHCAs across 455 hospitals using the GWTG-R data between 2003 and 2010. These investigators found that most IHCAs occur in the ICU (59%), and noted a temporal increase in the percentage of cases of IHCA occurring in the ICU.[34] This trend may represent an improvement in the ability to identify and move patients at highest risk to monitored units.[34] These investigators found that patients in the ICU were more likely to have a shockable rhythm (21% vs 17%, $P<.001$), and found that patients on monitored units had higher rates of survival than those on nonmonitored units.[34] Specifically, patients on telemetry units showed the highest survival rate (19.3%), followed by ICUs (14%) and unmonitored units (10.6%).[34] The lower survival of patients in the ICU compared with those on telemetry units is likely explained by the higher acuity and more critical nature of patients in the ICU.

Regional Variation

Variations in outcomes also exist at the regional level. In a national study of 838,465 patients with IHCA between 2003 and 2011, Kolte and colleagues[35] found significant regional variation in outcomes, with the lowest rate of survival among patients in the northeast versus the Midwest, south, and west (20.7%, 27.7%, 24.3%, 26.2% respectively).

Arrest Incidence

Interestingly, there may be an inverse relationship between a hospital's incidence of cardiac arrest and survival. In a national study of more than 100,000 IHCA cases across 358 hospitals, Chen and colleagues[25] found that hospitals with the lowest incidence of IHCA had the highest survival rates, even after controlling for case mix. However, hospital factors were attributed in part to some of this effect.[25] The factors causing the most significant shift were geographic region and the nurse-to-patient ratio.[25] Findings from this study suggest that the lower incidence of cardiac arrest in some hospitals may result from better overall quality of resuscitation care, including better prevention of IHCA. Findings also raise the importance of system factors such as nurse-to-patient ratio, which are associated with improved quality of care.

Time/Day, Nurse Staffing, and Resources

In addition, nurse staffing, time of day, and the day of the week have all been shown to affect outcomes significantly. Research continues to identify poorer outcomes for IHCA occurring on nights and weekends (off shifts). Perbedy and colleagues[36] noted that IHCAs occurring on off shifts were less likely to be monitored (74% vs 77%) and that the initial rhythm was less likely to be shockable (19.6% vs 22.9%). These investigators also found that rates of ROSC, survival to discharge, and good neurologic outcomes were significantly worse for IHCA occurring on off shifts.[36] Similar outcomes have been identified in more recent studies. Patel and colleagues[20] found that patients experiencing IHCA on off shifts were significantly less likely to receive early defibrillation (for shockable rhythms) or epinephrine administration (for nonshockable rhythms). Other studies exploring differences in survival on weekdays versus nights or weekends continue to identify suboptimal outcomes on off shifts.[10,17,23] Several factors often associated with off shifts may contribute to disparate outcomes, such as a higher percentage of inexperienced staff, fewer resource and support personnel, the impact of shift work (such as increased staff fatigue), and increased nurse-to-patient ratios.[10,23,36]

TREATMENTS FACTORS
Prevention

As stated previously, the prevention of IHCA is a primary goal. Identifying patients at the highest risk and placing them on an appropriately monitored unit can assist with earlier identification and management of deterioration. There is some evidence that IHCAs are increasingly occurring on monitored units,[34] suggesting potential improvements in prevention. However, moving patients to a monitored unit alone may be insufficient. Optimal outcomes require that providers are skilled at identifying early signs of deterioration and that systems to support optimal processes are in place. Cardiac arrest occurring in the ICU is often presumed to be nonpreventable because of the constant monitoring that occurs in this environment; however, Moskowitz and colleagues[37] identified several factors contributing to IHCA occurring in the ICU that may be amenable to further prevention strategies. The top factors included delayed response to deterioration, missed or incorrect diagnosis, delayed communication with the attending physician, delayed escalation of care, and administration of sedatives or narcotics for clinical deterioration.[37] Findings from this study highlight the need for ongoing efforts to optimize prevention of IHCA. Further research is needed to better understand the factors most amenable to prevention and to evaluate the effectiveness of strategies to optimize related outcomes.

Initial Treatment

When IHCA does occur, treatment based on the best available evidence is critical. The AHA has recently released updated guidelines for adult basic and advanced life support, which focuses on initial treatment and postresuscitation care, and includes the addition of recovery and survivor support.[38,39] An in-depth review of the initial treatment guidelines is beyond the scope of this article; however, a brief review is provided later.

Immediate implementation of high-quality cardiopulmonary resuscitation (CPR) remains the mainstay of initial resuscitation efforts. The emphasis of chest compressions is on pushing hard and fast at a rate of 100 to 120 beats/min, and at a depth of at least 50mm (2″) for adult patients, while allowing complete recoil.[39] Monitoring for an interruption in chest compressions has emerged as an important contributor to optimal resuscitation quality and outcomes.[24] Early defibrillation and epinephrine administration are also critical during the initial phases of resuscitation, including defibrillation within 2 minutes for shockable rhythms, administration of epinephrine within 5 minutes for nonshockable rhythms, administration of epinephrine after initial defibrillation attempts have failed for shockable rhythms, and continued administration of epinephrine every 3 to 5 minutes for cardiac arrest.[39]

Important updates in the 2020 guidelines include a shift to prioritizing peripheral intravenous versus intraosseous (IO) placement based on several recent studies that have brought the safety and efficacy of the IO route into question.[40] The recommendations suggest that the IO route may be used if unable to obtain peripheral intravenous (IV) access or if attempts are not feasible. The 2020 guidelines also include specialized management of certain conditions, such as electrolyte abnormalities, pregnancy, and after cardiac surgery.[39]

Postresuscitation Care

In addition to initial resuscitation, high-quality postresuscitation care is essential to optimizing outcomes for IHCA. The 2020 AHA guidelines provide updated recommendations for postresuscitation care. The updated algorithm focuses on blood pressure management, monitoring and treatment of seizures, and targeted temperature management (TTM).[38,39]

TTM to treat unwitnessed OHCA has been in use for more than a decade to improve neurologic outcomes for comatose patients and has been widely supported. During a juried evaluation of available evidence related to hypothermia for critical illness such as cardiac arrest, 5 intensive care professional societies strongly recommended TTM of 32°C to 34°C for unconscious patients with OHCA with VF or pulseless VT after the restoration of spontaneous circulation.[41] Since that time, increasing evidence has also been reported that suggests 34°C to 36°C may be the optimal temperature target. In 2017, Kirkegaard and colleagues[42] led an international, randomized clinical superiority trial that included 10 ICUs in 10 university hospitals across Europe. This study included 355 patients with OHCA who received a TTM of 33°C for either 24 hours or 48 hours. The group with longer TTM had more favorable outcomes (less mortality and better neurologic survival) but had more adverse events.[42] Kleissner and colleagues[43] recently evaluated the differences between the 2 temperature ranges. The investigators noted mixed results in their study of 175 patients with OHCA in 1 international ICU. Results showed no differences in 6-month survival or neurologic recovery between a historical cohort treated with 32°C to 35°C versus a prospective cohort treated with 34°C to 36°C.[43] The lower-temperature group had lower cerebral metabolism but also had higher complications.[43]

Because of initial research indicating an improvement in neurologic function in out-of-hospital arrests, TTM has been trialed for IHCA.[17] Results have been mixed. Some studies have failed to show a survival benefit or improved neurologic function among patients with IHCA.[17,44] In a cohort study of 1524 hypothermia-treated IHCAs that were propensity matched to 3714 normothermia patients with IHCA, Chan and colleagues[44] found that those treated with hypothermia had lower rates of both in-hospitable survival and neurologic survival.

More recently, Lascarrou and colleagues[45] conducted a randomized control trial to compare TTM at 33°C for 24 hours versus targeted normothermia among survivors of cardiac arrest with a nonshockable rhythm. Both patients with IHCA and those with OHCA were included. Patients who received TTM at 33°C showed improvement in survival and neurologic recovery, and outcomes were similar among patients with IHCA and OHCA.[45] To date, no randomized controlled trials have been published on outcomes of TTM among IHCA survivors with shockable rhythms. Based on the evolving evidence, TTM continues to be recommended as an important component of high-quality postarrest care.

Specific Recommendations for Postresuscitation Care

Specific recommendations for postresuscitation care include the following:

- Maintenance of normotension. The goal of hemodynamic management in patients after cardiac arrest is to ensure optimal perfusion of organ and brain tissue.[46] Specific targets include a systolic blood pressure greater than 90 mm Hg and a mean arterial pressure greater than 65 mm Hg.[47] Treatment of hypotension includes the administration of crystalloid fluid resuscitation, vasopressors, and or inotropes.
- Maintenance of normoxemia. The goal of oxygen management is to avoid hypoxia, which can contribute to ischemia, and hyperoxia, which can contribute to reperfusion injury and resultant neuronal death.[46] Before the ability to accurately measure oxygen levels, the highest available oxygen concentration should be

delivered. Once accurate oxygen measurement is available, oxygen delivery should be titrated to an SpO_2 of 92% to 98%.[47]

- Maintenance of normocarbia. Maintenance of normocarbia is important in optimizing cerebral perfusion. Hypercarbia can lead to cerebral vasodilatation, potentially contributing to increased intracranial pressure and decreased cerebral perfusion, whereas hypocarbia leads to cerebral vasoconstriction, which may result in decreased cerebral blood flow and decreased cerebral perfusion. In general, $PaCO_2$ levels between 35 mm Hg and 45 mm Hg should be targeted.[47]

- TTM. TTM is intended to reduce cerebral metabolism and decrease the risk of reperfusion injury. Current guidelines for the postresuscitation management of comatose patients following IHCA include the provision of TTM of 32°C to 36°C for 24 hours using an advanced cooling device with a feedback loop.[47]

- Seizure management. Up to 22% of comatose patients following cardiac arrest experience seizure, and nonconvulsive status epilepticus may contribute to ongoing coma.[46] For this reason, comatose patients following cardiac arrest should receive continuous electroencephalogram (EEG) monitoring to facilitate the detection and treatment of seizures.[47]

Emerging Considerations

In addition, the 2020 AHA guidelines recognize several emerging areas for which more research is needed. These areas include the use of arterial blood pressure tracings to guide CPR among patients with an arterial line already in place, evaluation of the safety and efficacy of IO devices, identification of populations most likely to benefit from extracorporeal membrane oxygenation, considerations for the use of point-of-care ultrasonography, evaluation of outcomes of TTM versus normothermia and optimal rewarming protocols, and the use of naloxone in opioid-associated cardiac arrest.

SUMMARY

Outcomes of IHCA are poor but have continued to improve over time. The wide-scale collection of standardized data on IHCA has supported the expansion of research evidence focused on IHCA, and subsequent quality improvement efforts focused on translating evidence into practice. Together, these efforts have contributed to improvements in outcomes for patients with IHCA. Although improving, wide variations in outcomes are attributed in part to differences in the overall quality of resuscitation care. The optimal quality of resuscitation care depends on the ability to apply the best available evidence to practice. As the providers with the closest proximity to the bedside, critical care nurses play an essential role in delivering the best evidence-based practices for patients with IHCA. This article provides an overview of the evidence related to IHCA, providing a foundation for critical care nursing practice related to the care of this population.

CLINICS CARE POINTS

- The primary focus for improvement of outcomes related to IHCA is on prevention. This focus includes identifying patients at highest risk for cardiac arrest, ensuring that high-risk patients are cared for in a monitored unit at a level of care appropriate to the patient, and ensuring that nurses and other providers are skilled in identifying and managing signs of clinical deterioration.

- Patients showing signs of clinical deterioration should receive appropriate escalation of care, including communication with advanced practice providers and the attending physician, and implementation of treatments to reverse the underlying cause of deterioration.

- Immediate, high-quality CPR remains the mainstay of resuscitation, including chest compressions that are hard and fast with a depth of at least 50 mm (2″) in adult patients, a rate of 100 to 120 beats/min, and allowing full chest recoil between compressions.
- Monitoring for the quality of chest compressions has emerged as an important factor in improving outcomes of IHCA.
- The peripheral IV is preferred to IO access. IO access is acceptable if attempts at peripheral IV access fail or if attempts at peripheral IV access are not feasible.
- Patients with IHCA should receive early treatment, including:
  o Defibrillation within 2 minutes for shockable rhythms
  o Administration of epinephrine within 5 minutes for nonshockable rhythms
- Patients should receive high-quality postresuscitation care, including:
  o Maintenance of normoxemia (Spo_2 92%–98%), normocarbia ($Paco_2$ 35–45 mm Hg), and normotension (systolic blood pressure >90 mm Hg, mean arteria pressure >65 mm Hg)
  o Implementation of TTM to achieve a target temperature of 32°C to 36°C for 24 hours, and monitoring and management of seizures, including continuous EEG in comatose patients following ROSC.
- The provision of meticulous critical care nursing is an important predictor of outcomes for patients with IHCA.

DISCLOSURE

The authors have nothing to disclose.

REFERENCES

1. American Heart Association. AHA statistical update: heart disease and stroke statistics - 2018 update. Circulation 2018;137(12):e67–492.
2. Murphy S, Xu J, Kochanek K, et al. Mortality in the United States, 2017. NCHS Data Brief 2018;328:1–8.
3. Neumar R. Doubling cardiac arrest survival by 2020: achieving the American heart association impact goal. Circulation 2016;134:2037–9.
4. McNally B, Robb R, Mehta M, et al. Out-of-hospital cardiac arrest surveillance - cardiac arrest registry to enhance survival (CARES), United States, October, 1, 2005 - december 31, 2010. MMWR Morb Mortal Wkly Rep 2011;60(8):1–19.
5. Anderson L, Holmberg M, Berg K, et al. In-hospital cardiac arrest: a review. JAMA 2019;1200–10.
6. Moskowitz A, Holmberg M, Donnino M, et al. In-hospital cardiac arrest - are we overlooking a key distinction? Curr Opin Crit Care 2018;24:151–7.
7. Sinha S, Sukul DL, Polavarapu V, et al. Identifying important gaps in randomized control trials of adult cardiac arrest treatments: a systematic review of the literature. Circ Cardiovasc Qual Outcomes 2016;9:749–56.
8. Institute of Medicine. Strategies to improve cardiac arrest survival: a time to act. Washington, DC: The National Academies Press; 2015.
9. Kronick S, Kurz M, Lin S, et al. Part 4: systems of care and continuous quality improvement: 2015 American Heart Association guidelines update for cardiopulmonary resuscitation and emergency cardiovascular care. Circulation 2015;132:S394–413.
10. American Heart Association. Heart disease and stroke statistics - 2020 update: a report from the American Heart Association. Circulation 2020;141:e139–469.

11. Nolan J, Berg R, Anderson L, et al. Cardiac arrest and cardiopulmonary resuscitation outcome reports: update of the Utstein resuscitation template for in-hospital cardiac arrest. Circulation 2019;140:e746–57.

12. Chan P, McNally B, Tang F, et al. Recent trends in survival from out-of-hospital cardiac arrest in the United States. Circulation 2014;130:1876–82.

13. American Heart Association. Get with the guidelines - resuscitation overview. 2020. Available at: https://www.heart.org/en/professional/quality-improvement/get-with-the-guidelines/get-with-the-guidelines-resuscitation/get-with-the-guidelines-resuscitation-overview. Accessed December 5, 2020.

14. Attin M, Tucker R, Carey M. In-hospital cardiac arrest: an update on pulseless electrical activity and asystole. Crit Care Nurse Clin North Am 2016;28:387–97.

15. Merchant R, Yang L, Becker L, et al. Incidence of treated cardiac arrest in hospitalized patients in the United States. Crit Care Med 2011;39:2401–6.

16. Holmberg M, Ross C, Fitzmaurice G, et al. Annual incidence of adult and pediatric in-hospital cardiac arrest in the United States. Circ Cardiovasc Qual Outcomes 2019;12.

17. Nichol G, Huszti E, Kim F, et al. Does induction of hypothermia improve outcomes after in-hospital cardiac arrest? Resuscitation 2013;84:620–5.

18. Chan P, Tang Y. Risk-standardizing rates of return of spontaneous circulation for in-hospital cardiac arrest to facilitate hospital comparisons. J Am Heart Assoc 2020;7(9):e014837.

19. Meaney P, Nadkarni V, Kern K, et al. Rhythms and outcomes of adult in-hospital cardiac arrest. Crit Care Med 2010;38:101–8.

20. Patel K, Spertus J, Khariton Y, et al. Association between prompt defibrillation and epinephrine treatment with long-term survival after in-hospital cardiac arrest. Circulation 2018;137:2041–51.

21. Morrison L, Neumar R, Zimmerman J, et al. Strategies for improving survival after in-hospital cardiac arrest in the United States: 2013 Consensus Recommendations. Circulation 2013;127:1538–63.

22. Schluep M, Gravesteijn B, Stolker R, et al. One-year survival after in-hospital cardiac arrest: a systematic review and meta-analysis. Resuscitation 2018;132:90–100.

23. Merchant R, Berg R, Yang L, et al. Hospital variation in survival after in-hospital cardiac arrest. J Am Heart Assoc 2014;3:1–8.

24. Chan P, Krein S, Tang F, et al. Resuscitation practices associated with survival after in-hospital cardiac arrest: a nationwide survey. JAMA Cardiol 2016;1:189–97.

25. Chen L, Nallamothu B, Spertus J, et al. Association between a hospital's rate of cardiac arrest incidence and survival. JAMA Intern Med 2013;173:1186–94.

26. Girotra S, Nallamothu B, Spertus J, et al. Trends in survival after in-hospital cardiac arrest. N Engl J Med 2012;367:1912–20.

27. Chan P, Berg R, Spertus J, et al. Risk-standardized survival for in-hospital cardiac arrest to facilitate hospital comparisons. J Am Coll Cardiol 2013;62:601–9.

28. Chan P, Nallamothu B, Krumholz HS, et al. Long-term outcomes in elderly survivors of in-hospital cardiac arrest. N Engl J Med 2013;368:1019–26.

29. Lee J, Chan P, Bradley S, et al. Temporal changes in the racial gap in survival after in-hospital cardiac arrest. JAMA Cardiol 2017;2:976–84.

30. Chen N, Callaway C, Guyette F, et al. Arrest etiology among patients resuscitated from cardiac arrest. Resuscitation 2018;130:33–40.

31. Wallmuller C, Meron G, Kurkciyan I, et al. Causes of in-hospital cardiac arrest and influence on outcome. Resuscitation 2012;83:1206–11.

32. Fehnel C, Trepman A, Steele D, et al. Survival after in-hospital cardiac arrest among cerebrovascular disease patients. J Clin Neurosci 2018;54:1–13.

33. Donnino M, Salciccioli J, Howell M, et al. Time to administration of epinephrine and outcome after in-hospital cardiac arrest with non-shockable rhythms: retrospective analysis of large in-hospital registry data. BMJ 2014;348:1–9.

34. Perman S, Stanton E, Soar J, et al. Location of in-hospital cardiac arrest in the United States: variability in event rate and outcomes. J Am Heart Assoc 2016; 5:1–7.

35. Kolte D, Khera S, Aronow W, et al. Regional variation in the incidence and outcomes of in-hospital cardiac arrest. Circulation 2015;131:1415–25.

36. Peberdy MA, Ornato J, Larkin GL, et al. Survival from in-hospital cardiac arrest during nights and weekends. JAMA 2008;299:785–92.

37. Moskowitz A, Berg K, Cocchi M, et al. Cardiac arrest in the intensive care unit: an assessment of preventability. Resuscitation 2019;145:15–20.

38. Merchant R, Topjian A, Panchal A, et al. Part 1: executive summary: American Heart Association guidelines for cardiopulmonary resuscitation and emergency cardiovascular care. Circulation 2020;14:S337–57.

39. Panchal A, Bartos J, Cabanas J, et al. Part 3: adult basic and advanced life support. Circulation 2020;142:S366–468.

40. Granfeldt A, Avis S, Lind PH, et al. Intravenous vs intraosseous administration of drugs during cardiac arrest. Resuscitation 2020;149:150–7.

41. Nunnally M, Jaeschke R, Bellingan G, et al. Targeted temperature management in critical care: a report and recommendations from five professional societies. Crit Care Med 2011;39:1113–25.

42. Kirkegaard H, Søreide E, de Haas I, et al. Targeted temperature management for 48 vs 24 hours and neurologic outcome after out-of-hospital cardiac arrest: a randomized control trial. JAMA 2017;318:341–50.

43. Kleissner M, Sramko M, Kautzner J, et al. Mid-term clinical outcomes of out-of-hospital cardiac arrest patients treated with targeted temperature management at 34-36 C versus 32-34 C. Heart Lung 2019;8:273–7.

44. Chan P, Berg R, Tang Y, et al. Association between therapeutic hypothermia and survival after in-hospital cardiac arrest. JAMA 2016;316:1375–82.

45. Lascarrou JB, Merdji H, Le Gouge A, et al. Targeted temperature management for cardiac arrest with non-shockable rhythm. N Engl J Med 2019;381:2327–37.

46. Clifton CW, Donnino M, Fink E, et al. Part 8: post-cardiac arrest care: 2015 American Heart Association guidelines update for cardiopulmonary resuscitation and emergency cardiovascular care. Circulation 2015;132:S465–82.

47. American Heart Association. Highlights of the 2020 American heart association guidelines for CPR and ECC. Dallas: American Heart Association. 2020.

The Role of Tele-Critical Care in Rescue and Resuscitation

Fiona A. Winterbottom, DNP, MSN, APRN, ACNS-BC, ACHPN, CCRN[1]

KEYWORDS

- Tele-ICU • Tele-critical care • Rapid response • Resuscitation

KEY POINTS

- Tele-critical care (TCC) has many novel applications that can be used for patient safety.
- The combination of TCC, the electronic medical record, and other technologies provides opportunities for innovative care delivery systems.
- TCC was used in creative ways during the COVID-19 pandemic.

Tele-critical care (TCC) can be described as a health care delivery model that connects medical information through advanced pathways, such as audio-video interfaces, machine learning, risk prediction algorithms, smart alarms, artificial intelligence, and physiologic sensing devices.[1,2] A combination of TCC and the electronic medical record (EMR) allows for expansion of critical care services and expertise beyond the walls of the intensive care unit (ICU). The role of TCC in rescue and recovery is growing especially where mature Rapid Response Systems (RRS) exist. A combination of TCC and the EMR allows for expansion of critical care services and expertise beyond the walls of the ICU. TCC can leverage other technologies that cohort patients into virtual units and create computer-generated lists that allow for patient screening. Virtual units and watchlists can be combined using TCC and the EMR to provide remote surveillance of patients who are at high risk of clinical deterioration. Over the past decade, these technologies have advanced, as have the clinicians who use the tools. This article demonstrates interoperability of TCC, the EMR, and clinical implementation science in development of rescue and resuscitation systems.

OCHSNER HEALTH

Ochsner Health is Louisiana's largest nonprofit, academic, health care system with 40 owned, managed, and affiliated hospitals. Ochsner TCC is part of CareConnect 360,

The author has nothing to disclose.

Critical Care Medicine, Ochsner Health, Pulmonary Critical Care, Ochsner Medical Center, 1514 Jefferson Highway, New Orleans, LA, USA

[1] Present address: Pulmonary Department, Ochsner Medical Center, 9th Floor Clinic, New Orleans, LA 70121, USA

E-mail address: Fwinterbottom@Ochsner.org

Ochsner's telehealth program. The TCC hub is located at the Ochsner Health Center–Elmwood; Ochsner Medical Center–New Orleans is a 700-bed acute care Magnet-recognized academic hospital, and Ochsner Medical Center–West Bank is a 180-bed acute care community facility. These facilities are all located close to the Mississippi River, within 10 miles of New Orleans city center.

TCC and the EMR were implemented at Ochsner Health in 2012. The Ochsner TCC hub monitors approximately 200 beds and is staffed by nurses 24 hours per day, with remote intensivists providing additional overnight coverage. Ochsner Health RRS is staffed differently in academic and community facilities depending on local resource availability and infrastructure. Each site uses standardized tools within the TCC and EMR platforms to support surveillance, rescue, and resuscitation of patients experiencing clinical deterioration. Case examples from the Ochsner Health TCC are used throughout this article to illustrate the application of concepts in practice.

TELE-CRITICAL CARE OVERVIEW

TCC can be described as connected services from a remote site to a recipient at a local site where physical care is provided.[2] The traditional TCC model uses audiovisual communication systems to support the treatment of critically ill patients.[1] Original models were designed to bridge staffing shortages of intensivists and critical care nurses as the demand for critical care services and patient complexity increased.[1] TCC models can be characterized in the 3 following ways: (1) A centralized hub-and-spoke model where a single remote center (hub) provides continuous 24/7 TCC services to multiple locations (spokes); (2) a decentralized, point-to-point episodic model; and (3) a hybrid model that combines the 2 modalities.[2,3] Several interprofessional staffing models exist that include nurses, physicians, advanced practice providers, pharmacists, respiratory therapists, and other allied health professionals.[2,3] Most traditional TCC models include hardwired bedside equipment that is permanently fixed in place and a mechanism to request TCC services from inside the ICU room.[2,3] Rolling carts, workstations, and portable devices may also be used in conjunction with hardwired equipment to offer additional mobile, flexible solutions. **Fig. 1** shows a TCC workstation, and **Fig. 2** shows a view of the patient bed from the perspective of the TCC staff.

TCC is continuing to evolve and is expanding to support any location where critical care is delivered.[2] Although historically used to support care in the ICU, novel uses of TCC outside ICU include logistic centers, emergency departments (ED), general wards, war zones, disaster settings, and pandemics.[2] TCC rapidly provides expertise and evaluation at the point of care using an assortment of encrypted, HIPAA-compliant wireless technologies to connect mobile devices, cameras, and computers in hospitals, homes, and other environments.[2,3] TCC provides surveillance and expertise in multiple clinical contexts through purposeful goal-directed data collection, interpretation, synthesis, and analysis of patients using clinical decision support, monitoring, predicative analytics, and risk stratification.[2,3] TCC supports the development, implementation, and monitoring of evidence-based practices and protocols. TCC also supports the collection and analysis of data on quality metrics that can be used to inform performance improvement and resource stewardship.[2,3]

TCC consultation can be made by request of bedside staff or by automated alert to the remote monitoring center. In rooms that have hardwired equipment, a call button on the wall of the patient's room can be pressed by bedside staff to call for assistance from TCC. Examples of this type of call include monitoring of procedures, documentation of timeouts, or for communication about transport. In transport situations, TCC

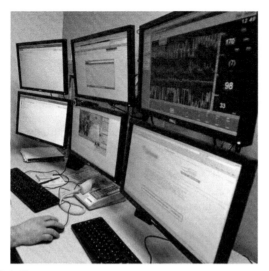

Fig. 1. A TCC workstation.

is informed about patients leaving the unit, which allows TCC staff to increase monitoring of the nurse's other patients when they are off the unit. Alternatively, TCC can initiate a consult when they see abnormal trends or alarms, such as in cardiac arrest situations. Mobile carts and tablets have request and drop-in capabilities, or telephone systems can be used for communication.

TELE-CRITICAL CARE SERVICES OUTSIDE INTENSIVE CARE UNIT

Critical care services are often required beyond the walls of the ICU. ED frequently admit and hold patients who need ICU care.[4,5] Studies demonstrate that ICU patients

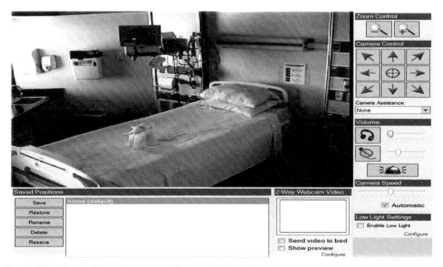

Fig. 2. The view of a patient room from a TCC workstation.

who spend hours in the ED waiting for a bed have worse outcomes than those imme-diately admitted to an ICU bed.[4,5] TCC monitoring of ICU patients in the ED has been shown to decrease mortality and reduce ICU utilization.[5] Collaboration between ED, ICU, and TCC provides opportunities to improve equitable care delivery during pe-riods of surge and overcrowding.[4,6,7]

RRS can also use TCC to bridge gaps in care delivery systems where critical care is needed outside of the ICU. Many centers have developed innovative RRS that support patients transferring into the ICU, direct admissions, procedural areas, and ED. Enhanced surveillance from TCC and RRS combined with other technological solu-tions, such as machine learning, risk prediction algorithms, early warning scores (EWS), artificial intelligence, and physiologic sensing devices, may help identify pa-tients experiencing clinical deterioration earlier and reduce preventable mortality through earlier intervention.[8]

A study in a children's hospital found that TCC expedited intensivist bedside response times and allowed for delivery of life-saving interventions in the initial critical minutes of severe clinical deterioration.[8] In the study, TCC intensivist response times averaged 2.6 minutes versus bedside arrival times of 3.7 minutes, thus expediting time to intervention by an expert resuscitator.[8] Another children's hospital compared in-person response times at a TCC hub with pediatric intensivist support to RRS and code teams at spoke satellite facilities.[9] The TCC model was found to be reliable, effi-cient, and effective with median response times in both groups of 7 minutes for RRS activations and 1.5 minutes for codes.[9] In the Telemedicine Resuscitation and Arrest Trial, TCC use was assessed in care of patients with out-of-hospital cardiac arrest (OHCA) and severe sepsis. In the study, an on-call TCC team supported 3 ED to care for critically ill patients through remote access to a telemedicine cart, EMR ac-cess, and protocolized workflows. Mean time from OHCA TCC consult request to TCC connection was 3.7 minutes with a mean call duration of 71.7 minutes, and mean time from sepsis TCC consult request to TCC connection was 8.4 minutes with a mean call duration on 61.5 minutes.[10,11] The study showed that it was opera-tionally feasible for the TCC team to assist with ventilator management, medication management, and device troubleshooting during the consultation, as well as interact-ing with families in the busy ED.[10,11] Another multicenter study investigated the perceived utility of TCC as expert resuscitators during in-hospital cardiac arrest. Pos-itive perceptions of TCC as a "copilot" emerged from the study with smaller commu-nity hospitals perceiving the most benefit from TCC support.[12] These studies provide evidence that TCC can be adapted to a variety of health care environments to provide rapid expert critical care support to bedside staff.

CASE PRESENTATION: TELE-CRITICAL CARE AND CARDIOPULMONARY ARREST

In 2013, TCC nurses at Ochsner Health identified an opportunity to assist nurses at the bedside during cardiopulmonary arrest situations. Because most of the nurses that worked in TCC also worked at the bedside, they recognized that their colleagues had difficulty documenting in the EMR during emergency situations. Given the clinical realities, bedside nurses would often need to prioritize patient care, leaving documen-tation until a later time. This led to delays in documentation, decreased accuracy of data capture, additional stressors for bedside staff, and increased overtime. The TCC nurses asked if they could pilot an intervention whereby they would help docu-ment the emergency events. In addition to documentation, TCC nurses helped to ensure optimal timing of interventions, monitoring, and documentation of data on key performance indicators. TCC nurses have been able to assist in many cardiopulmonary arrest cases (**Fig. 3**). This nurse-driven solution has led to other interventions, such as documentation of procedural timeouts, such as central line placement, arterial lines, intubation, paracentesis, and thoracentesis. The TCC nurses also help disseminate best practices during procedures and ensure lines, drains, and airways are properly documented in the EMR.

INTEROPERABILITY AND CLINICAL IMPLEMENTATION SCIENCE

TCC leverages interoperable technology together with implementation science to drive improvements in quality and safety outcomes. Interoperability describes how equipment or groups interface to advance effective care delivery. Interoperability of technology, such as machine learning, risk prediction algorithms, EWS, artificial intelligence, physiologic sensing devices, and clinician workflows, is needed to optimize care delivery systems to prevent adverse events. The tools can only be effective if they are used by bedside clinicians to optimize care. Implementation science involves examining barriers and facilitators to uptake of evidence-based practices and identifying the most effective strategies for translating evidence into practice.[13] Examining barriers and facilitators that slow or expedite uptake of proven evidence-based care practices is a necessary component of interoperability. A systematic review by the National Heart, Lung, and Blood Institute Implementation Science Work Group found that barriers to clinician guideline uptake included time constraints, staffing limitations, timing, skepticism, knowledge, and clinician age.[13] The work group found that facilitators to clinician guideline uptake included format, resources, end-user/stakeholder involvement, leadership support, scope of implementation, organizational culture, teamwork, and electronic systems.[13] Strategies involving audit, feedback, and educational outreach have been found to be efficacious in process of care and clinical outcome improvement, whereas reminders and incentives have demonstrated limited effectiveness.[13] These barriers and facilitators are particularly important to consider as technology is integrated into clinical care and adherence to best practices, clinical outcomes, and fiscal impact is evaluated.[13] TCC leverages interoperable technologies and implementation science to optimize patient care.

One clinical care practice that may be greatly influenced by technology is routine vital sign monitoring.[14,15] Routine vital sign monitoring is a basic nursing function of patient care that has remained unchanged for years and yet has limited studies to

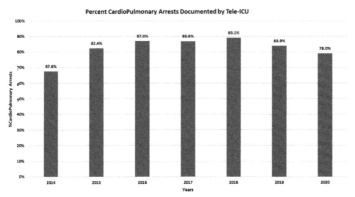

Fig. 3. Percentage of cardiopulmonary arrests documented by TCC nurses. Numerator = number of arrests documented by TCC nurses. Denominator = total number of cardiopulmonary arrests documented in the EMR in units with TCC monitoring.

demonstrate effectiveness in prevention of clinical deterioration and adverse events on general wards.[14,15] Novel technologies are providing opportunities for continuous vital sign monitoring that may reduce unexpected clinical deterioration and prevent adverse events.[14,15] A systematic review searched for studies comparing effectiveness of intermittent and continuous monitoring of vital signs on general wards.[14] Effectiveness was defined as prevention of adverse events, cardiac arrests, and transfers to ICU. Many diverse vital sign surveillance practices were identified in the study, such as combinations of automated, semiautomated, and manual monitoring; however, limited studies addressing the effectiveness of vital sign monitoring were found.[14] The investigators concluded that neither an intermittent nor a continuous vital sign monitoring strategy could be recommended as effective in prevention of clinical deterioration and adverse events on general wards because of heterogeneity and insufficiency of existing evidence.[14] Another evolving method for prevention of clinical deterioration and adverse events on general wards is through the use of composite EWS. These EWS are derived from vital signs and can be scored on paper or in the EMR. The goal of these scores is to alert clinicians to vital sign derangement and promote early recognition of clinical deterioration using a protocolized approach to care escalation.[15] A study examining adherence to vital sign safety protocols on general wards using a modified early warning score (MEWS) found a 49% adherence rate to a care escalation protocol.[15] The investigators determined that inappropriate protocol adherence could negatively impact nurses' responses to critical situations, including clinical deterioration, and indicated that missed assessment and documentation of vital signs may contribute to negative outcomes.[15] This evidence suggests that barriers to optimal detection and prevention of clinical deterioration include insufficient frequency of vital sign monitoring, failure to identify concerning trends, and failure to implement early interventions. TCC can help to overcome these barriers by leveraging wearable technologies that facilitate continuous vital sign monitoring in connection with technology that allows for more sophisticated detection of concerning trends, and connection with appropriate clinical decision support technology.

New technologies, such as continuous surveillance and wearable sensors, may offer solutions to overcome barriers to vital sign monitoring and protocol adherence while improving patient safety.[16,17] Several approved wearable sensors are available on the market.[14] Although there are limitations to each wearable device, the potential to improve utilization and adoption exists if clinician and patient stakeholders are engaged in product development.[16,17] Another benefit of wearable technology is the ability to monitor respiratory rate. Despite the knowledge that respiratory rate predicts clinical deterioration, it is often inaccurately measured and poorly reported.[18–20] In a study on alert thresholds, respiratory rate had the highest positive predictive value for clinical deterioration, whereas heart rate had the lowest.[18] Although limited evidence exists to support the use of wearable devices for critically ill patients, these emerging technologies hold potential to improve patient safety for patients at hospital and at home. Many hospitals, including Ochsner Health, are piloting these novel technologies to promote safe patient care while reducing the discomfort of bulky monitoring devices that disrupt circadian rhythms with noise and alerts. Because wearable devices and other novel technologies allow for continuous surveillance and alerts, there is capability to notify clinicians of concerning clinical trends in real-time. These physiologic sensing devices can prompt clinicians to initiate actions using clinical decision support, such as machine learning, risk prediction algorithms, EWS, and artificial intelligence.[21,22]

Although real-time clinical decision support is desirable, there is a need to consider the volume of alarms sent to clinicians to prevent alarm fatigue.[21,22] A systematic review demonstrated that intensive care nurses perceived that alarms were burdensome and interfered with patient care, which reduced trust in alarm systems.[22] Nurses felt overburdened by excessive, continuous alarms, and operation of advanced medical equipment that took time away from patient care.[22] The study concluded that alarm fatigue could have serious consequences for patients and nursing personnel; therefore, alarm management strategies and mechanisms for measuring alarm fatigue should be implemented.[22] Implementation science strategies, such as end-user/stakeholder involvement, cognitive staffing limitations, organizational culture, and teamwork, could be helpful in developing successful and sustainable systems of care. In addition to delivery of alerts, it is necessary to consider what should be done with alert information received by the clinician and what escalation should occur. Initially, the clinician must decide if each alarm is clinically relevant or insignificant before taking any action, and subsequently decide on a specific intervention. One study reported that an ICU nurse might receive 150 to 400 alarms per patient per shift.[22] A study on nurses' decision making related to clinical deterioration found that barriers to escalation included balancing alert uncertainty/validity and complex team dynamics on wards, which led to workarounds.[23] An MEWS protocol compliance study that looked at how nurses responded to abnormal vital signs showed that protocol compliance decreased as risk score increased.[15] The reasons for noncompliance with such protocols could be due to inability to manage the increased vital sign monitoring, cognitive workload, lack of time to document interventions, technology acceptance, or other simultaneous competing priorities. TCC can play a role in optimizing patient outcomes through external cognitive support for tracking, trending, and responding to alerts without the distractions experienced by clinicians, such as call bells, rounds, medication administration, and patient transport. TCC responsibilities include efficient information gathering through use of high-technological audio-video, electronic, and telecommunication tools that provide rapid surveillance of multiple patients at once as well as efficient movement from 1 patient to another without physical obstacles or geographic distance.[3]

Solutions to the complexities of clinical deterioration may be mitigated through clinical leadership, teamwork, and technology. Dedicated RRS can become the action arm for alerts received by TCC from physiologic sensing devices, machine learning, risk prediction algorithms, EWS, and artificial intelligence. RRS are clinical experts who are focused on clinical deterioration and can support clinical staff.[24] Barriers to successful implementation of RRS include medical hierarchy, unclear calling criteria, alarm fatigue, and lack of hospital system integration.[24] Facilitators of successful RRS include defined leadership structures, interprofessional collaboration and training, clear protocols, feedback, and evaluation.[24] Tiered RRS offer another method for proactive assessment, urgent clinical review, and peer support while providing a clear delineated pathway with criteria for escalation.[25,26] Tiered systems provide escalation protocols with defined criteria that aligns with clinician's scope of practice.[26] Tiered protocols may include nurse-to-charge nurse escalation, charge nurse-to-primary team escalation for clinical review and then further escalation for RRS and critical care evaluation.[26]

CASE PRESENTATION: TELE-CRITICAL CARE, RAPID RESPONSE SYSTEMS, AND COVID-19

In 2017, a 24/7 proactive rapid response nurse (RRN) program was implemented to reduce adverse events and cardiac arrest outside ICU. The Ochsner Institutional Review Board approved the RRN study. The program combined novel artificial intelligence alerts, expert nurse rounding, interprofessional training, closed-loop communication, quality improvement, and targeted outcome measurement to offer a customized approach to reduce preventable deaths and resuscitation events outside the ICU. In the first year after the program implementation, a 74% reduction in cardiopulmonary arrests outside the ICU and a 30% reduction in cardiopulmonary arrest inside ICU were seen. In 2019, a rapid response respiratory therapist was added to the team after cardiopulmonary arrest case reviews showed that clinical deterioration was often due to respiratory pathologic condition. This became the Ochsner Medical Center RRS.

During March 2020, there was a surge of patients admitted to the New Orleans area hospitals because of the COVID-19 pandemic. One positive outcome of the crisis was the opportunity for innovative use of technology. TCC was expanded across Ochsner hospitals to expand virtual support for delivery of critical care from 200 beds to 461 beds. Twenty-six TCC carts were also deployed to areas such as endoscopy and recovery rooms to support patients and redeployed noncritical care staff in delivery of ICU level care. TCC was placed on computer terminals within ICUs and other areas to facilitate patient assessment remotely. This decreased the need for frequent entry into patient rooms, decreased personal protective equipment (PPE) use, and reduced unnecessary staff exposure to the virus.[27] Multiple vendor platforms and devices were adapted to provide remote monitoring through computers, smartphones, and tablets. Wearable device technology and artificial intelligence alerts were scaled across Ochsner hospitals so that the technologies could use unvalidated EMR vital sign data to trigger clinical deterioration alerts for risk-stratification assessment. Ochsner Medical Center's proactive 24/7 RRS used existing technologies plus TCC for surveillance of patient surge demands outside the ICU. A TCC station was set up in the RRS office so patients could be connected to the team with audio-visual communication. This increased team efficiency and reduced time spent moving geographically from 1 patient to another. Continuous patient assessment using TCC technology reduced the time and frequency of patient room entry, thereby decreasing use of PPE, limiting staff exposure to the virus, while still promoting patient safety.[27] This strategy adapted existing TCC and RRS models to meet the demands of the rapidly changing environment.

Standardized written order guidelines expanded RRN scope of practice to consult critical care providers for patients at high risk of deterioration and to initiate orders for diagnostics, imaging, and medications, such as arterial blood gases, X rays, oxygen, and intravenous fluids. Patients with higher acuity than usual were transferred out of the ICU. These patients remained at high risk of deterioration and ICU readmission and were monitored by the RRS. During the COVID-19 pandemic, the RRS acted as a mobile ICU team that could triage patients, initiate clinical interventions, and follow up on patients transferred out of the ICU. This model provided hospitalwide support for overextended bedside clinicians. Average monthly RRN activity is routinely tracked and trended. Data from 2019 were compared with RRN activity for March 2020 during the peak of the COVID-19 pandemic in New Orleans. There was an increase in high-risk screening (97%), RRN consults (375%), rapid responses (22%), intubations (220%), and transfers to the ICU (83%). During the same time, the number of COVID-19–positive patients went from 0 to 340, and the number of ventilated patients went from 27 to 121 in a 10-day period. Increases in RRN consults indicate that the RRS was heavily used as a support system during the pandemic and demonstrate that floor nurses and other staff felt comfortable calling for help. RRN activity validates the ability of the proactive team to flex the capacity to meet the COVID-19 patient surge.

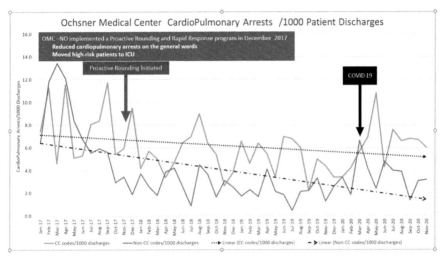

Fig. 4. . Ochsner Medical Center rate of critical care (CC) and non-CC cardiopulmonary arrests per 1000 patient discharges between January 2017 and November 2020. OMC, Ochsner Medical Center; NO, New Orleans.

As patient volume increased across New Orleans, community hospitals were also affected by the COVID-19 pandemic. The Ochsner Medical Center West Bank community hospital ICU team was able to rapidly initiate a proactive 24/7 RRN program using the standardized risk prediction algorithms, EWS, orders, workflows, and documentation used at Ochsner Medical Center. Ochsner Medical Center–West Bank hospital also used TCC access and mobile carts to monitor patients, decrease PPE usage, and mitigate staff expose to the virus. **Figs. 4–6** demonstrate the resuscitation outcomes from Ochsner Medical Center and Ochsner Westbank Medical Center before and during the COVID-19 pandemic.

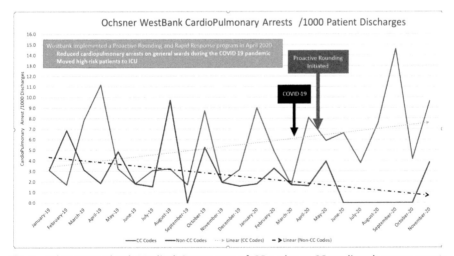

Fig. 5. Ochsner Westbank Medical Center rate of CC and non-CC cardiopulmonary arrests per 1000 patient discharges between January 2019 and November 2020.

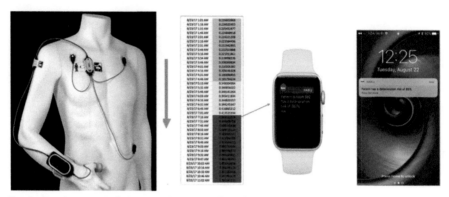

Fig. 6. Continuous vital sign monitoring and artificial intelligence alerts.

SUMMARY

TCC has many novel applications for patient safety. Combining TCC, audio-video interfaces, physiologic sensing devices, machine learning, risk prediction algorithms, smart alarms, and artificial intelligence expands critical care expertise beyond the walls of the ICU and offers opportunities to advance innovative patient care delivery systems. The potential benefits of TCC was demonstrated within 1 health system during the COVID-19 pandemic in 2020.

ACKNOWLEDGMENTS

The author would like to thank Ochsner Tele-ICU, Ochsner Medical Center, and Ochsner Westbank leaders and rapid response teams for their contributions.

REFERENCES

1. Khurrum M, Asmar S, Joseph B. Telemedicine in the ICU: innovation in the critical care process. J Intensive Care Med 2020. 0885066620968518.
2. Subramanian S, et al. Tele-critical care: an update from the Society of Critical Care Medicine Tele-ICU Committee. Read Online Crit Care Med Soy Cril Care Mee 2020;48(4):553–61.
3. Rincon TA, Henneman E. An introduction to nursing surveillance in the tele-ICU. Nursing2019 Crit Care 2018;13(2):42–6.
4. Markus S. Effect of emergency department and ICU occupancy on admission decisions and outcomes for critically ill patients: Mathews KS, Durst MS, Vargas-Torres C, et al. Critical Care Medicine. 2018;46(5):720-727. J Emerg Med 2018;55(3):451–2.
5. Kadar RB, et al. Impact of telemonitoring of critically ill emergency department patients awaiting ICU transfer. Crit Care Med 2019;47(9):1201–7.
6. Lilly CM, Mullen M. Critical care surge management. Crit Care Med 2019;47(9): 1271–3.
7. Subbe CP, et al. Quality metrics for the evaluation of rapid response systems: proceedings from the third international consensus conference on rapid response systems. Resuscitation 2019;141:1–12.
8. Robison J, Nicholas B. A more rapid, rapid response. Pediatr Crit Care Med 2016;17(9):871–5.

9. Berrens ZJ, et al. Efficacy and safety of pediatric critical care physician telemedicine involvement in rapid response team and code response in a satellite facility. Pediatr Crit Care Med 2019;20(2):172.

10. Agarwal AK, et al. Telemedicine REsuscitation and Arrest Trial (TREAT): a feasibility study of real-time provider-to-provider telemedicine for the care of critically ill patients. Heliyon 2016;2(4):e00099.

11. Nadar M, et al. Impact of synchronous telemedicine models on clinical outcomes in pediatric acute care settings: a systematic review. Pediatr Crit Care Med 2018; 19(12):e662.

12. Peltan ID, et al. Acceptability and perceived utility of telemedical consultation during cardiac arrest resuscitation. A multicenter survey. Ann Am Thorac Soc 2020;17(3):321–8, e671.

13. Chan WV, et al. ACC/AHA special report: clinical practice guideline implementation strategies: a summary of systematic reviews by the NHLBI implementation science work group: a report of the American College of Cardiology/American Heart Association Task Force on clinical practice guidelines. J Am Coll Cardiol 2017;69(8):1076–92.

14. Cardona-Morrell M, et al. Effectiveness of continuous or intermittent vital signs monitoring in preventing adverse events on general wards: a systematic review and meta-analysis. Int J Clin Pract 2016;70(10):806–24.

15. Eddahchouri Y, et al. Low compliance to a vital sign safety protocol on general hospital wards: a retrospective cohort study. Int J Nurs Stud 2020;115: 103849.

16. Weenk M, et al. Wireless and continuous monitoring of vital signs in patients at the general ward. Resuscitation 2019;136:47–53.

17. Joshi M, et al. Wearable sensors to improve detection of patient deterioration. Expert Rev Med Devices 2019;16(2):145–54.

18. Keim-Malpass J, et al. Towards development of alert thresholds for clinical deterioration using continuous predictive analytics monitoring. J Clin Monit Comput 2019;1–8.

19. Fieselmann JF, et al. Respiratory rate predicts cardiopulmonary arrest for internal medicine inpatients. J Gen Intern Med 1993;8(7):354–60.

20. Sprogis SK, et al. Physiological antecedents and ward clinician responses before medical emergency team activation. Crit Care resuscitation 2017;19(1):50–6.

21. Churpek MM, et al. Multicenter comparison of machine learning methods and conventional regression for predicting clinical deterioration on the wards. Crit Care Med 2016;44(2):368.

22. Lewandowska K, et al. Impact of alarm fatigue on the work of nurses in an intensive care environment—a systematic review. Int J Environ Res Public Health 2020;17(22):8409.

23. Bingham G, et al. The pre-medical emergency team response: nurses' decision-making escalating deterioration to treating teams using urgent review criteria. J Adv Nurs 2020;76(8):2171–81.

24. Olsen SL, et al. Succeeding with rapid response systems–a never-ending process: a systematic review of how health-care professionals perceive facilitators and barriers within the limbs of the RRS. Resuscitation 2019;144:75–90.

25. Aneman A, et al. Characteristics and outcomes of patients admitted to ICU following activation of the medical emergency team: impact of introducing a two-tier response system. Crit Care Med 2015;43(4):765–73.

26. Bingham G, et al. Clinical review criteria and medical emergency teams: evaluating a two-tier rapid response system. Crit Care Resuscitation 2015; 17(3):167.
27. Rathod N, et al. e-ICU's/Tele ICU's, it's role, advantages over manual ICU's and shortcomings in the current perspective of covid-19 pandemic: a critical review. IJCRR 2020;12(13).

Moving?

Make sure your subscription moves with you!

To notify us of your new address, find your **Clinics Account Number** (located on your mailing label above your name), and contact customer service at:

Email: journalscustomerservice-usa@elsevier.com

800-654-2452 (subscribers in the U.S. & Canada)
314-447-8871 (subscribers outside of the U.S. & Canada)

Fax number: 314-447-8029

Elsevier Health Sciences Division
Subscription Customer Service
3251 Riverport Lane
Maryland Heights, MO 63043

*To ensure uninterrupted delivery of your subscription, please notify us at least 4 weeks in advance of move.